# DIABETIC HIGH FIBER COOKBOOK

• • • • •

## MARY JANE FINSAND

FOREWORD BY JAMES D. HEALY, M.D., F.A.A.P.

Sterling Publishing Co., Inc.   New York

**Other Books by Mary Jane Finsand**
*Caring & Cooking for the Hyperactive Child*
*The Complete Diabetic Cookbook*
*Diabetic Candy, Cookie & Dessert Cookbook*
*The Diabetic Chocolate Cookbook*

EDITED BY VILMA LIACOURAS CHANTILES

**Library of Congress Cataloging in Publication Data**
Finsand, Mary Jane.
  Diabetic high fiber cookbook.

  Includes index.
    1. Diabetes—Diet therapy—Recipes.
2. High-fiber diet—Recipes.  I. Title.
RC662.F566   1985      641.5′637      85-9876
ISBN 0-8069-5584-8
ISBN 0-8069-6228-3 (pbk.)

Published by Sterling Publishing Co., Inc.
Two Park Avenue, New York, N.Y. 10016
Distributed in Australia by Capricorn Book Co. Pty. Ltd.
Unit 5C1 Lincoln St., Lane Cove, N.S.W. 2066
Distributed in the United Kingdom by Blandford Press
Link House, West Street, Poole, Dorset BH15 1LL, England
Distributed in Canada by Oak Tree Press Ltd.
% Canadian Manda Group, P.O. Box 920, Station U
Toronto, Ontario, Canada M8Z 5P9
*Manufactured in the United States of America*

# Contents

# Foreword

Considerable research and the trend towards natural foods have made the public aware of the need for more dietary fiber to maintain healthy bodies. The diabetic's need to reduce sugar intake, balance the required food nutrients and eat a wide variety of delicious foods has always been difficult. Adding fiber to an already restricted diet can appear to be a difficult problem. This *Diabetic High Fiber Cookbook* will help diabetics and other readers on restricted diets follow their doctor's recommendations and still eat a wide variety of delectable foods that *they* like to eat.

This cookbook is an excellent companion to Mary Jane Finsand's previous books, *The Complete Diabetic Cookbook, Diabetic Candy, Cookie & Dessert Cookbook* and *The Diabetic Chocolate Cookbook*. All recipes in Mary Jane's diabetic cookbooks are complete with calories and food exchange information to allow users to regulate food intake within medically prescribed recommendations.

I believe that anyone—including diabetics and other people on restricted diets—will use this cookbook frequently as a kitchen reference for preparing delicious high-fiber dishes and meals. The recipes, food exchanges and calorie data should complement your doctor's recommendations and assist you in enjoying your meals. Please share this cookbook with your doctor, pharmacist, hospital dietitian and staff members of your diabetic organization. I am confident that they will confirm my high recommendation.

James D. Healy, M.D., F.A.A.P.

# *Preface*

I know what you are thinking. In my earlier books, I said I wanted to help remove the word "restricted" from your diabetic diet, and now I tell you to add fiber. Is this a contradiction? Not at all. I wrote this book because I am convinced it is a good idea to increase the dietary fiber in your diet. And believe me, you will not need to change your eating habits. I will not take away your favorite foods nor will you need to change your diabetic exchanges or calories.

I will, however, show you how to increase your fiber intake simply by creating new recipes for you. I am not the only one interested in the addition of fiber to your diet. You will find many new recipes created for you by some American food manufacturers, by diabetics and a chapter—Sausages—written for you by my husband, Louis Finsand.

It would be absurd to say that everything you eat should have fiber in it or that this book has all the answers. But it is important to know what foods have fiber so that you can make the right choices yourself.

I hope you enjoy this cookbook as much as *The Complete Diabetic Cookbook, Diabetic Candy, Cookie & Dessert Cookbook* and *The Diabetic Chocolate Cookbook*.

Mary Jane Finsand

# Introduction

## Fiber & Your Diet

Many words have been written about fiber and the positive effects it has in the diets of diabetics. We are not going to rehash all this information. Instead, we provide a short review of fiber and then get right to the nitty-gritty of how to increase the fiber content in your diet.

## What Is Fiber?

Dietary fiber is found primarily in the nondigestible substances of plants. In the past, fiber has been referred to as *bulk* or *roughage*—meaning the residue remaining after digestion and absorption of food. Dietary fiber helps satisfy the appetite, aids the digestive system and helps in eliminating wastes regularly. Fiber helps with the formation of bulk and the absorption of water, a process that moves wastes through the digestive tract, decreasing the inner pressure on the colon. Fiber also aids in controlling blood sugar levels. A low-fiber diet, however, forms less residue. Buildups of wastes often occur in the intestine and colon, causing discomfort and constipation.

Dietary fiber includes the following components:

* *Cellulose*—found in fruits, vegetables, whole grain cereals and bran or bran products.
* *Lignin*—found in whole grain cereals, vegetables and fruits.
* *Hemicellulose*—found in whole grain cereals, vegetables and fruits.
* *Pentosan*—found in whole grain cereals, legumes, seeds and nuts, cabbage and fruits.
* *Gum*—found in beans, oats and oat bran.
* *Pectin*—found in apples and white membrane of citrus fruits.

## How Do I Increase Fiber in My Diet?

We are sure you are interested in ways to improve your diet by adding more fiber. To show how you can increase fiber in your diet, let's use an average lunch as an example.

## LUNCH

2 meat exchanges
2 bread exchanges
1 vegetable exchange
1 fruit exchange
1 milk exchange
1 fat exchange

| LOW-FIBER | HIGH-FIBER |
|---|---|
| 1 slice cold meat | 1 slice cold meat |
| 1 slice cheese | 1 slice cheese |
| 2 slices white bread | 2 slices whole wheat bread |
| 1 c. (250 mL) cooked summer squash | ½ c. (250 mL) cooked broccoli |
| ½ small banana | 10 strawberries |
| 1 c. (250 mL) milk | 1 c. (250 mL) milk |
| 1 t. (5 mL) mayonnaise | 1 t. (5 mL) mayonnaise |

At first glance, it seems we made no great changes. But look at the difference when we list the fiber content of the lunch. (The cold meat, cheese, milk and the mayonnaise are the same for both lunches, so we will not consider them.)

| FOOD | FIBER CONTENT | FOOD | FIBER CONTENT |
|---|---|---|---|
| 2 slices white bread | 1.2g | 2 slices whole wheat bread | 3.8g |
| 1 c. (250 mL) summer squash | 1.6g | ½ c. (250 mL) cooked broccoli | 3.1g |
| ½ small banana | 0.9g | 10 strawberries | 2.1g |
| **Total** | 3.7g | | 9.0g |

By a simple change you have more than doubled the fiber content in your lunch without changing the exchanges or the calories. Through the recipes in this book, you will easily be able to add the extra needed fiber to your diet. And *no, you will not have to count the grams of fiber*.

## How Much Fiber Is Enough?

Although there is no recommended daily amount, experts generally advise 35 to 40 grams of fiber per day for the average adult. The average adult eats daily about 15 to 20 grams of fiber. For you to determine the amount of extra fiber you need, it is important to begin by consulting your doctor or diet counsellor and ask if you should increase your dietary fiber every day. If the answer is affirmative, increase your fiber consumption by adding more complex carbohydrates (including legumes, whole grain products, such as breads and cereals), fruits and vegetables (raw, whenever possible). And remember to drink plenty of fluids when you add fiber to your diet. If you don't drink enough liquids, constipation can occur. You should be drinking at least eight or more glasses of water every day.

Remember, a good diet contains only what the body needs. And the body needs adequate, not excessive, amounts of vitamins, minerals, proteins, fats and carbohydrates, some of which should be high in fiber.

If you have any questions about your diet, please feel free to write to us.

Darlene Duke, R.N.
Hattie Middleton, R.D.
Schoitz Diabetes Education Resource Center
Schoitz Medical Center
2101 Kimbel Avenue
Waterloo, IA 50702

# Using the Recipes for Your Diet

Read the recipes carefully, then assemble all equipment and ingredients. Use standard measuring equipment (whether metric or customary, be sure to measure accurately). Remember, these recipes are good for everyone, not just the diabetic.

**Customary Terms**

| | |
|---|---|
| t. | teaspoon |
| T. | tablespoon |
| c. | cup |
| pkg. | package |
| pt. | pint |
| qt. | quart |
| oz. | ounce |
| lb. | pound |
| °F | degrees Fahrenheit |
| in. | inch |

**Metric Symbols**

| | |
|---|---|
| mL | millilitre |
| L | litre |
| g | gram |
| kg | kilogram |
| °C | degrees Celsius |
| mm | millimetre |
| cm | centimetre |

# Breakfast

## Crispy Baked French Toast

| | | |
|---|---|---|
| 2 | eggs, well-beaten | 2 |
| ½ c. | 2% milk | 125 mL |
| ½ t. | salt | 2 mL |
| ½ t. | vanilla | 2 mL |
| 6 slices | Oroweat Northridge bread | 6 slices |
| 1 c. | Stone-Buhr bran flakes | 125 mL |
| ¼ c. | margarine, melted | 60 mL |

Combine eggs, milk, salt and vanilla in shallow dish or pan. Dip bread in egg mixture, turning once; allow time for both sides to absorb liquid. Coat evenly with bran flakes and place in a single layer on a well-greased baking sheet. Drizzle with the margarine. Bake at 450 °F (230 °C) for about 10 minutes or until crisp and browned. Serve warm.

**Yield:** 6 servings
**Exchange, 1 serving:** 1½ bread, 2 fat
**Calories, 1 serving:** 192

*With the compliments of Arnold Foods Company, Inc.*

## Apricot Morning Drink

| | | |
|---|---|---|
| 16-oz. can | Featherweight water pack apricot halves | 454-g can |
| 1½ c. | skim milk | 375 mL |
| 3 | eggs | 3 |
| 1 t. | vanilla extract | 5 mL |
| ½ t. | Featherweight liquid sweetener | 2 mL |
| | ground cinnamon | |

Combine all ingredients except the cinnamon in a blender and cover. Blend at medium speed 30 seconds. Pour into glasses and sprinkle apricot drink with cinnamon.

**Yield:** 3 servings
**Exchange, 1 serving:** 1 fruit, 1 high-fat meat, ½ nonfat milk
**Calories, 1 serving:** 191

*Based on a recipe from Featherweight Brand Foods.*

## Broiled Grapefruit

A simple, but often forgotten, breakfast starter.

| | | |
|---|---|---|
| 1 | *grapefruit* | 1 |
| ½ t. | *butter* | 2 mL |
| 1 t. | *granulated sugar replacement* | 5 mL |
| dash | *ground cinnamon* | dash |
| dash | *ground or grated nutmeg* | dash |

Cut grapefruit in half crosswise. Loosen sections with a sharp knife or grapefruit spoon. Place ¼ t. (1 mL) butter in middle of each half. Sprinkle each half with ½ t. (2 mL) granulated sugar replacement, cinnamon and nutmeg. Broil 4 in. (10 cm) from heat for 6 to 8 minutes. Serve hot.
**Yield:** 2 servings
**Exchange, 1 serving:** 1 fruit, ½ fat
**Calories, 1 serving:** 60

## Citrus Cup

| | | |
|---|---|---|
| 4 | *oranges* | 4 |
| ½ c. | *fresh shredded coconut, chopped* | 125 mL |
| 8-oz. can | *Featherweight grapefruit segments, drained* | 227-g can |
| 8-oz. can | *Featherweight pineapple, drained and cut into eighths* | 227-g can |

Cut off top third of oranges. Scoop out pulp, slice into pieces and put into a bowl. Set orange shells in custard cups. Reserve 1 T. (15 mL) coconut. Add remaining coconut, grapefruit and pineapple to orange pieces; toss gently. Spoon fruit into orange shells. Top with reserved coconut.
**Yield:** 4 servings
**Exchange, 1 serving:** 4 fruit, ½ fat
**Calories, 1 serving:** 192

*Based on a recipe from Featherweight Brand Foods.*

## Baked Apples

| | | |
|---|---|---|
| 4 medium | *Rome apples* | 4 medium |
| ¼ c. | *walnuts, chopped* | 60 mL |
| ¼ c. | *raisins* | 60 mL |
| ¼ c. | *Health Valley Orangeola cereal with almonds and dates* | 60 mL |
| ¼ t. | *ground cinnamon* | 1 mL |

Wash and core apples. Place in ovenproof dish. In small bowl, mix together the remaining ingredients. Divide into 4 portions and fill each apple hole with 1 portion. Cover and bake at 350 °F (175 °C) for 1 hour.
**Yield:** 4 servings
**Exchange, 1 serving:** ½ bread, 2 fruit, 1 fat
**Calories, 1 serving:** 165

*From Health Valley Foods.*

## Baked Apple Fritters

| 1 c. | Health Valley honey graham crackers, crushed into crumbs | 200 mL |
|------|-----------------------------------------------------------|--------|
| 1 t. | ground cinnamon | 5 mL |
| 2 large | pippin apples, cored and each sliced into 4 rings | 2 large |
| 4 T. | lemon juice | 60 mL |

Combine graham cracker crumbs with cinnamon. Dip apple slices in lemon juice and then graham cracker crumbs. Coat well on both sides. Place on greased cookie sheet. Bake at 400 °F (200 °C) for 15 to 20 minutes.
**Yield:** 4 servings
**Exchange, 1 serving:** 2 bread, 1 fruit
**Calories, 1 serving:** 170

*From Health Valley Foods.*

## Mixed Fruit Cocktail

| 8-oz. can | Featherweight sliced peaches, drained; reserve 1 T. (15 mL) liquid | 227-g can |
|-----------|-------------------------------------------------------------------|-----------|
| 8-oz. can | Featherweight pear halves, drained and cut in quarters | 227-g can |
| 8-oz. can | Featherweight sliced pineapple, drained and cut in quarters | 227-g can |
| 8-oz. can | Featherweight purple plums, drained, pitted and cut in halves | 227-g can |
| ½ c. | Featherweight apricot preserves | 125 mL |

Combine drained fruit in a bowl. Mix preserves and reserved peach liquid in a small saucepan; heat thoroughly. Pour over fruit and stir.
**Yield:** 4 servings
**Exchange, 1 serving:** 3 fruit
**Calories, 1 serving:** 117

*Based on a recipe from Featherweight Brand Foods.*

## Scrambled Eggs Primavera

| | | |
|---|---|---|
| 2 T. | Mazola corn oil | 30 mL |
| 1 c. | zucchini, chopped | 250 mL |
| ½ c. | mushrooms, sliced | 125 mL |
| ¼ c. | green onion, thinly sliced | 60 mL |
| 4 | eggs, lightly beaten with fork | 4 |
| dash | dried basil | dash |
| 4 | English muffins, split and toasted | 4 |
| 1 | tomato, chopped | 1 |
| 1 T. | parsley, chopped | 15 mL |

In a skillet, heat oil over medium-high heat. Add next 3 ingredients. Cook and stir for 2 minutes or until zucchini is crisp-tender. Reduce heat to medium low. Add eggs and basil. Cook and stir for 3 to 4 minutes or until eggs are set. Spoon onto muffin halves. Garnish with tomato and parsley.

**Yield:** 4 servings

**Exchange, 1 serving:** 2 bread, 1 low-fat milk, 1 vegetable

**Calories, 1 serving:** 290

*"A Diet for the Young at Heart" by Mazola.*

## Italian Scrambled Eggs

| | | |
|---|---|---|
| 1 small | butternut squash, thinly sliced | 1 small |
| 1 small | onion, thinly sliced | 1 small |
| 3 T. | butter | 45 mL |
| 1 c. | meatless spaghetti sauce | 250 mL |
| | salt and pepper to taste | |
| 4 | large eggs | 4 |
| 2 T. | water | 30 mL |

In a medium skillet, lightly sauté squash and onion in 1 T. (15 mL) of the butter until onion is translucent. Add spaghetti sauce and season with salt and pepper; simmer 5 minutes and set aside. Beat together the eggs and water. In a large skillet, scramble eggs in remaining butter. Serve eggs topped with vegetable-sauce mixture.

**Yield:** 4 servings

**Exchange, 1 serving:** 1 bread, 1 vegetable, 1 medium-fat meat, 1 fat

**Calories, 1 serving:** 213

## Wheat-Germ Waffles

| 1¾ c. | sifted Stone-Buhr all-purpose flour | 440 mL |
| 3 T. | granulated sugar replacement | 45 mL |
| 2 t. | baking powder | 10 mL |
| | salt | |
| ⅔ c. | Stone-Buhr wheat germ | 160 mL |
| 2 c. | skim milk | 500 mL |
| ⅓ c. | vegetable oil | 90 mL |
| 2 | eggs, separated | 2 |

Sift together the flour, sugar replacement, baking powder and salt. Add wheat germ and stir to mix. Combine and beat milk, oil and egg yolks. Add to flour mixture; beat until smooth. In another bowl, beat egg whites until stiff but not dry. Fold into batter. Bake in preheated waffle iron.

**Yield:** 5 servings
**Exchange, 1 serving:** 2 bread, 1 low-fat milk
**Calories, 1 serving:** 261

*Based on a recipe of Arnold Foods Company, Inc.*

## Sesame Whole Wheat Pancakes

| 1 c. | Stone-Buhr whole wheat pancake mix | 250 mL |
| 1¼ c. | skim milk | 310 mL |
| 1 | egg | 1 |
| ⅓ c. | Stone-Buhr sesame seeds, toasted | 90 mL |

Combine the pancake mix, milk and egg. Pour a little less than ¼ c. (60 mL) batter for each pancake onto a lightly greased griddle. Immediately sprinkle each pancake with about 2 t. (10 mL) toasted sesame seeds. Turn pancake when bubbles appear on the surface.

**Yield:** 6 servings
**Exchange, 1 serving:** 1 bread, 1 medium-fat meat
**Calories, 1 serving:** 150

*With the compliments of Arnold Foods Company, Inc.*

## Prune Streusel Coffeecake

| | | |
|---|---|---|
| 3 T. | all-purpose flour | 45 mL |
| 2 T. | granulated brown sugar replacement | 30 mL |
| 2 t. | ground cinnamon | 10 mL |
| ½ c. | Bran Buds cereal | 125 mL |
| 3 T. | margarine, softened | 45 mL |
| 1 c. | all-purpose flour | 250 mL |
| ¾ t. | baking powder | 4 mL |
| ¾ t. | baking soda | 4 mL |
| ½ t. | salt | 2 mL |
| ½ t. | ground cinnamon | 2 mL |
| ¾ c. | Bran Buds cereal | 190 mL |
| ½ c. | margarine, softened | 125 mL |
| 2 T. | granulated sugar replacement | 30 mL |
| 2 | eggs | 2 |
| 1 c. | plain low-fat yogurt | 250 mL |
| ½ c. | pitted prunes, finely cut | 125 mL |

For the topping: measure the first 5 ingredients into a small mixing bowl. Mix with fork or fingers until crumbly. Set aside.

For the cake: stir together 1 c. (250 mL) flour, baking powder, baking soda, salt, cinnamon and ¾ c. (190 mL) cereal. Set aside. In a large bowl, beat ½ c. (125 mL) margarine and sugar replacement until well blended. Add eggs. Beat well. Stir in yogurt. Add flour mixture, mixing thoroughly. Spread half the batter evenly in greased 9-inch (23-cm)-square baking pan. Sprinkle evenly over the batter, half the prunes and then, half the topping. Spread remaining batter over the top and sprinkle batter with the remaining prunes and topping mixture. Bake at 350 °F (175 °C) about 40 minutes or until done. Serve warm.

**Yield:** 16 servings
**Exchange, 1 serving:** 1 bread, ⅔ low-fat milk, ½ fat
**Calories, 1 serving:** 180

*Adapted from a recipe from Kellogg's Test Kitchens.*

## Spicy Prune Bread

| | | |
|---|---|---|
| 2 c. | all-purpose flour, sifted | 500 mL |
| 2½ t. | baking powder | 12 mL |
| ½ t. | baking soda | 2 mL |
| 1 t. | salt | 5 mL |
| 1 t. | ground cinnamon | 5 mL |
| ½ t. | ground or grated nutmeg | 2 mL |
| ¼ t. | ground cloves | 1 mL |

| | | |
|---|---|---|
| 1 c. | oatmeal | 250 mL |
| 1¼ c. | buttermilk | 310 mL |
| 2 T. | vegetable oil | 30 mL |
| 1 c. | prunes, cooked, drained, pitted and diced | 250 mL |

Sift together the flour, baking powder, baking soda, salt, cinnamon, nutmeg and cloves. Stir in the oatmeal. Add buttermilk and oil; stir to completely blend. Fold in prunes. Spread into a well-greased 9 × 5-in. (23 × 13-cm) loaf pan. Bake at 350 °F (175 °C) for 1 hour or until done. Turn out on rack to cool.

**Yield:** 1 loaf or 16 servings
**Exchange, 1 serving:** 1 bread, ¼ fruit
**Calories, 1 serving:** 85

## Orangeola Bars

| | | |
|---|---|---|
| 1¼ c. | Health Valley Orangeola cereal | 310 mL |
| ¼ c. | Health Valley Sprouts 7 cereal | 60 mL |
| ⅓ c. | walnuts, finely ground | 90 mL |
| 2 T. | fresh or dried coconut, grated | 30 mL |
| dash | ground or grated nutmeg | dash |
| 2 T. | clover honey | 30 mL |
| ½ t. | vanilla | 2 mL |
| 2 | egg whites, beaten until stiff | 2 |

In a mixing bowl, combine cereals, nuts, coconut and nutmeg. Add honey and vanilla and mix thoroughly (it might be necessary to use your hands to do this). Then fold in egg whites and allow mixture to stand 2 to 3 minutes. Spread or press into greased 11 × 6½ × 2-in. (28 × 16.5 × 5-cm) baking pan. Bake in preheated 275 °F (135 °C) oven for 20 minutes. Remove from oven. Cut into 20 to 24 bars and transfer immediately to glass or china plate to cool.

**Yield:** 20 bars
**Exchange, 1 bar:** ⅔ bread
**Calories, 1 bar:** 50

*From Health Valley Foods.*

# Raisin Apple Spiral

| | | |
|---|---|---|
| 1 pkg. | active dry yeast | 1 pkg. |
| ¾ c. | milk, warmed | 190 mL |
| ¼ c. | margarine, softened | 60 mL |
| ½ t. | salt | 2 mL |
| 2¼ c. | all-purpose flour | 560 mL |
| 1 c. | wheat germ | 250 mL |
| 1 | egg | 1 |
| 1 recipe | Raisin Apple Filling (recipe follows) | 1 recipe |
| | vegetable oil for brushing dough | |
| 1 | egg | 1 |
| 1 T. | water | 15 mL |
| ⅓ c. | Powdered Sugar Replacement (recipe follows) | 90 mL |
| ¼ t. | orange rind, grated | 1 mL |
| 3 t. | orange juice | 15 mL |

In a large bowl, dissolve the yeast in warm milk. Add margarine and salt, stirring until margarine almost melts. Stir in 1 c. (250 mL) of the flour, wheat germ and egg. With an electric mixer, beat at medium speed for 2 minutes. Scrape bowl occasionally. With wooden spoon, gradually stir in just enough remaining flour to make a soft dough which leaves sides of bowl. Cover and allow to rise in warm, draft-free place about 1 hour or until doubled. Roll on floured board into a 24 × 4-in. (61 × 10-cm) strip. Spread the Raisin Apple Filling across middle of strip. To seal, lift dough and pinch lengthwise edges together with seam-side down, coil loosely, snail fashion. Place on greased baking sheet with space between to allow for rising. Brush dough lightly with oil. Cover and allow to rise about 1 hour or until doubled. Brush with 1 egg mixed with the water just before baking. Bake at 350 °F (175 °C) for 20 to 25 minutes until golden. Immediately remove from baking sheet. Cool slightly on rack. Combine powdered sugar replacement and orange rind and gradually add orange juice, beating until smooth. Drizzle on bread. Serve warm.

## RAISIN APPLE FILLING

| | | |
|---|---|---|
| 1 c. | apple, chopped | 250 mL |
| ½ c. | raisins | 125 mL |
| 2 T. | butter | 30 mL |
| ½ c. | walnuts, chopped | 125 mL |
| 2 T. | orange rind, grated | 30 mL |
| ¼ t. | ground cinnamon | 1 mL |
| ¼ t. | ground or grated nutmeg | 1 mL |
| dash | ground cloves | dash |
| dash | salt | dash |

Combine apple, raisins and butter in a small saucepan. Cover and simmer over low heat for 10 minutes. Remove from heat and stir in the remaining ingredients. Cool.
**Yield:** 1 coffee cake or 24 servings
**Exchange, 1 serving:** 1 bread, 1 fat
**Calories, 1 serving:** 112

# Powdered Sugar Replacement

| | | |
|---|---|---|
| 2 c. | *nonfat dry milk powder* | *500 mL* |
| 2 c. | *cornstarch* | *500 mL* |
| 1 c. | *granulated sugar replacement* | *250 mL* |

Combine all ingredients in food processor or blender. Whip until well blended into a powder.
**Yield:** 4 c. (1 kg)
**Exchange, 1 serving:** ¼ c. (60 mL): 1 bread or ½ nonfat milk, ½ bread
**Calories, 1 serving:** ¼ c. (60 mL): 81

*From* Diabetic Candy, Cookie & Dessert Cookbook
*(Sterling Publishing Co., Inc., 1982).*

# Raspberry Preserves

For this recipe, I substituted raspberries in Blueberry Preserves from *The Complete Diabetic Cookbook* (Sterling Publishing Co., 1980). Preserves can also be made with blueberries and strawberries.

| | | |
|---|---|---|
| 1 c. | *fresh or frozen unsweetened raspberries* | *250 mL* |
| 1 t. | *low-cal pectin* | *5 mL* |
| 1 t. | *granulated sugar replacement* | *5 mL* |

Place raspberries in top of double boiler and cook over boiling water until soft and juicy. As they cook, crush berries against sides of double boiler. Add pectin and sugar replacement. Blend in thoroughly. Cook until medium thick.
**Microwave:** Place raspberries in glass bowl. Cook on HIGH for 4 minutes until soft and juicy. Add pectin and sugar replacement. Blend thoroughly. Cook on HIGH for 30 seconds.
**Yield:** ⅔ c. (180 mL)
**Exchange, 2 T. (30 mL):** ⅕ fruit
**Calories, 2 T. (30 mL):** 7

## Orangey Pineapple-Nut Squares

Orangeola is a unique cereal made only by Health Valley. It gets its unusual flavor from sweet fruit and orange oil blended with oats.

| | | |
|---|---|---|
| 2 c. | Health Valley Orangeola cereal, finely crushed | 500 mL |
| ½ t. | ground ginger | 2 mL |
| 4 | egg yolks | 4 |
| 2 T. | safflower oil | 30 mL |
| ¾ c. | milk | 190 mL |
| ½ c. | pecans, chopped | 125 mL |
| 1 c. | unsweetened crushed pineapple, drained | 250 m |
| 4 | egg whites | 4 |

In a medium bowl, combine cereal and ginger. In a small bowl, beat egg yolks, then add oil and milk. Add to dry ingredients, then stir in nuts and pineapple. Beat egg whites until stiff and fold them into batter. Spoon batter into greased 8-in. (20-cm)-square baking pan. Bake in preheated 350 °F (175 °C) oven for 30 to 35 minutes, until toothpick inserted in middle comes out dry.

**Yield:** 9 servings
**Exchange, 1 serving:** 2 bread, 1 fruit, 3 fat
**Calories, 1 serving:** 315

*From Health Valley Foods.*

# Appetizers & Relishes

## Appetizer Meatballs

| ¾ lb. | ground beef | 375 g |
|---|---|---|
| ¼ lb. | ground pork | 125 g |
| ¾ c. | Stone-Buhr 4 grain cereal mates | 190 mL |
| ¼ c. | water chestnuts, finely chopped | 60 mL |
| ¼ t. | Worcestershire sauce | 1 mL |
| ½ c. | skim milk | 125 mL |
| ½ t. | garlic salt | 2 mL |
| few drops | Tabasco sauce | few drops |

Combine all ingredients and mix well. Shape into 75 small balls. In a nonstick pan, brown well over low heat. Place in chafing dish, add ½ c. (125 mL) warm water. Use toothpicks to serve.

**Yield:** 75 balls
**Exchange, 5 balls:** 1 medium-fat meat
**Calories, 5 balls:** 70

*With the compliments of Arnold Foods Company, Inc.*

## Sesame Cheese Balls

| 3-oz. pkg. | cream cheese, softened | 85-g pkg. |
|---|---|---|
| ¼ c. | blue cheese | 60 mL |
| ¼ c. | dried beef, minced | 60 mL |
| dash | cayenne pepper | dash |
| ¼ c. | Stone-Buhr sesame seeds, toasted | 60 mL |

Blend cheeses with dried beef and cayenne pepper. Shape into 20 small balls. Chill. Roll in sesame seeds.

**Yield:** 20 balls
**Exchange, 1 ball:** ½ fat
**Calories, 1 ball:** 23

*With the compliments of Arnold Foods Company, Inc.*

## Spinach Crescents

| | | |
|---|---|---|
| ½ c. | onion, finely chopped | 125 mL |
| 2 T. | cooking oil | 30 mL |
| 10-oz. pkg. | frozen chopped spinach, thawed and squeezed dry | 300-g pkg. |
| ¾ c. | Kretschmer regular wheat germ | 190 mL |
| ¾ c. | Parmesan cheese, grated | 190 mL |
| ½ c. | sour cream | 125 mL |
| ¼ c. | pine nuts | 60 mL |
| ½ t. | dried basil, crushed | 2 mL |
| ¼ t. | pepper | 1 mL |
| dash | salt | dash |
| 2 8-oz. pkg. | refrigerated crescent dinner rolls | 2 240-g pkg. |
| 1 | egg white, beaten | 1 |

Sauté onion in hot oil for 2 to 3 minutes until tender. Remove from heat. Add the remaining ingredients except crescent rolls and egg white. Mix the filling thoroughly. Separate crescent rolls into triangles. Cut each triangle in half lengthwise. Spread 1 T. (15 mL) of the filling, packed firmly, on each triangle. Roll up triangles, starting with the long end. Place on ungreased baking sheets. Brush with beaten egg white. Bake at 325 °F (165 °C) for 16 to 18 minutes until golden brown. Serve warm.

**Yield:** 32 appetizers
**Exchange, 1 appetizer:** ½ bread
**Calories, 1 appetizer:** 30

*With the courtesy of Kretschmer Wheat Germ/International Multifoods.*

## Spinach Dip

This dip has a very fresh flavor.

| | | |
|---|---|---|
| 10-oz. pkg. | spinach, chopped | 300-g pkg. |
| 2 T. | onions, chopped fine | 30 mL |
| 8 oz. | Dannon plain low-fat yogurt | 227 g |
| 1 T. | mayonnaise | 15 mL |
| ½ t. | salt | 2 mL |
| ¼ t. | black pepper | 1 mL |

Stir all ingredients together until well blended.
**Yield:** 1½ c. (375 mL)
**Exchange, ¼ c.** (60 mL): 1 fat
**Calories, ¼ c.** (60 mL): 48

# Cheese Wafers

| | | |
|---|---|---|
| ¾ c. | all-purpose flour | 190 mL |
| dash | cayenne pepper | dash |
| ¼ c. | sesame seeds, toasted | 60 mL |
| ½ c. | margarine, softened | 125 mL |
| 2 c. | sharp cheddar cheese, shredded | 500 mL |
| 1 c. | All-Bran or Bran Buds cereal | 250 mL |

Stir together flour and pepper. Set aside. Measure sesame seeds into small shallow bowl. Beat margarine and cheese until very light and fluffy. Stir in the cereal. Add flour mixture, mixing until well combined. Drop by rounded teaspoonfuls into sesame seeds. Coat evenly. Place on ungreased baking sheets. Flatten with fork that has been dipped in flour. Bake at 350 °F (175 °C) for 12 minutes or until lightly browned around edges. Remove immediately from baking sheets. Cool on wire racks.

**Yield:** 5 dozen wafers
**Exchange, 3 wafers:** ½ bread, 1 medium-fat meat
**Calories, 3 wafers:** 120

*From Kellogg's Test Kitchens.*

# Cheesy Herb Crackers

| | | |
|---|---|---|
| ⅔ c. | Kretschmer regular wheat germ | 165 mL |
| ⅓ c. | all-purpose flour | 90 mL |
| ½ t. | salt | 2 mL |
| ¾ c. | sharp cheddar cheese, grated | 190 mL |
| ¼ c. | margarine, softened | 60 mL |
| 1 T. | water | 15 mL |
| 2 T. | Kretschmer regular wheat germ | 30 mL |

Combine ⅔ c. (165 mL) wheat germ, flour and salt on waxed paper. Stir well to blend. Beat cheese and butter together until well-blended. Stir blended dry ingredients and water into cheese mixture. Mix well. Divide dough in half. Roll out each half on lightly floured, cloth-covered board to ⅛-in. (4-mm) thickness. Cut with 2-in. (5-cm) cutter that has been dipped in flour. Place on ungreased baking sheets. Sprinkle lightly with the additional 2 T. (30 mL) wheat germ. Bake at 350 °F (175 °C) for 8 to 10 minutes until very lightly browned. (Watch carefully to avoid overbrowning.) Remove from baking sheet. Cool on rack. Store in container with loosely fitting cover.

**Yield:** 4½ dozen crackers
**Exchange, 4 crackers:** 1 bread
**Calories, 4 crackers:** 68

*With the courtesy of Kretschmer Wheat Germ/International Multifoods.*

## Super Nachos

| | | |
|---|---|---|
| 8 oz. | firm tofu (bean curd), drained and cut into 1-in. (2.5-cm) cubes | 250 g |
| 1½ c. | water | 375 mL |
| ¼ c. | onion, chopped | 60 mL |
| 2 cloves | garlic, minced | 2 cloves |
| ¾ c. | Health Valley Bellissimo pasta sauce | 190 mL |
| dash | Tabasco sauce | dash |
| 6 oz. | ground beef | 180 g |
| ½ c. | mushrooms, chopped | 125 mL |
| 2 t. | chili powder | 10 mL |
| 1 t. | paprika | 5 mL |
| ½ t. | ground cumin | 2 mL |
| ½ t. | oregano | 2 mL |
| 1 t. | Health Valley Instead of Salt steak & hamburgers seasoning | 5 mL |
| 4 | corn tortillas | 4 |
| 4 oz. | cheddar cheese, grated | 120 g |
| 4 c. | lettuce, shredded | 1 L |
| 2 c. | tomatoes, diced | 500 mL |
| 1 c. | red pepper, chopped | 250 mL |
| 2 c. | green pepper, chopped picante sauce | 500 mL |

In a small saucepan, combine tofu, 1 c. (250 mL) of the water, 2 T. (30 mL) of the chopped onion and garlic. Bring to a boil. Reduce heat and simmer 10 minutes. Drain off the water. Put the mixture in food processor. Add pasta sauce and process until smooth. Season with Tabasco sauce. Set aside.

Meanwhile, brown meat with chopped mushrooms and 1 T. (15 mL) of the chopped onions. Add seasonings and remaining water and simmer for 10 minutes or until water evaporates. On baking sheet, arrange tortillas in a single layer. Bake at 450 °F (230 °C) until crisp, about 4 minutes on each side. Preheat broiler. Spread on each tortilla ¼ of the tofu mixture, then ¼ of the seasoned beef, then ¼ of the grated cheese. Broil until cheese is bubbly, about 5 minutes. Place each tortilla on a separate plate. Surround each tortilla with ¼ of each vegetable—lettuce, tomatoes, onions and red and green pepper. Serve picante sauce on the side.

**Yield:** 8 servings
**Exchange, 1 serving:** 1 bread, 1 high-fat meat
**Calories, 1 serving:** 180

*From Health Valley Foods.*

## Party Starters

| | | |
|---|---|---|
| 12 | large mushrooms | 12 |
| dash | lemon juice | dash |
| 2 T. | butter | 30 mL |
| 6½-oz. can | crab meat, drained and flaked | 195-g can |
| ¼ c. | La Choy water chestnuts, finely chopped | 60 mL |
| 1 T. | whole wheat bread crumbs | 15 mL |
| 1 T. | green onion, finely chopped | 15 mL |
| 1 t. | lemon juice | 5 mL |
| 1 t. | La Choy soy sauce | 5 mL |
| 1 T. | parsley, finely chopped | 15 mL |
| 1 | egg, slightly beaten | 1 |

Trim stems from mushrooms. Sprinkle caps with lemon juice. Finely chop the stems. Cook stems in butter for 2 minutes. Stir in the remaining ingredients, mixing well. Fill mushroom caps with mixture. Place in buttered 8-in. (20-cm)-square pan. Bake at 350 °F (175 °C) for 20 minutes. Serve hot.

**Yield:** 12 appetizers
**Exchange, 1 appetizer:** ½ lean meat
**Calories, 1 appetizer:** 29

*Adapted from a recipe from La Choy Food Products.*

## Hummus

| | | |
|---|---|---|
| 1½ c. | chick-peas, cooked and drained, (liquid reserved) | 375 mL |
| ½ c. | tahini (ground sesame seeds) | 125 mL |
| 1 clove | garlic | 1 clove |
| 3 T. | lemon juice | 45 mL |
| dash | cayenne pepper | dash |
| | chopped parsley for garnish | |

In the bowl of a blender, combine chick-peas, tahini, garlic and lemon juice. Process until smooth. If mixture is too thick to blend well, add 1 T. (15 mL) of reserved chick-pea cooking liquid. Sprinkle cayenne over top, garnish with parsley and serve with your favorite whole grain crackers.

**Yield:** 2 c. (500 mL)
**Exchange, ¼ c. (60 mL):** 1 medium-fat meat
**Calories, ¼ c. (60 mL):** 80

*From Health Valley Foods.*

## Wilted Relish

I like to serve this in a small serving bowl surrounded by Wasa crisp bread fiber. I cut each slice of the crisp bread into 6 cracker-type pieces.

| | | |
|---|---|---|
| 1 c. | cabbage, finely chopped | 250 mL |
| ½ c. | cucumber, finely chopped | 125 mL |
| ½ c. | onion, finely chopped | 125 mL |
| 3 T. | salt | 45 mL |

Combine ingredients in a bowl or jar. Cover tightly. Shake well to cover vegetables with salt. Marinate at room temperature for at least 24 hours; shake several times. Drop mixture into a fine mesh strainer and thoroughly rinse with cool water. Place in bowl, cover tightly and refrigerate until completely chilled.

**Yield:** 1½ c. (250 mL)
**Exchange:** negligible
**Calories:** negligible

## Crunchy Bran Jumble

| | | |
|---|---|---|
| 3 c. | Cracklin' Oat Bran cereal | 750 mL |
| 1 c. | salted peanuts | 250 mL |
| 1 c. | thin pretzel sticks | 250 mL |
| ⅓ c. | margarine, melted | 90 mL |
| 1 t. | Worcestershire sauce | 5 mL |
| ½ t. | seasoned salt | 2 mL |
| 1 T. | sesame seeds | 15 mL |

Measure cereal, peanuts and pretzels into 13 × 9 × 2-in. (33 × 23 × 5-cm) baking pan. Set aside. Stir together remaining ingredients. Pour over cereal mixture, stirring until well coated. Bake at 350 °F (175 °C) about 15 minutes. Do not stir. Cool in pan. Store in tightly covered container.

**Yield:** 5 cups (1¼ L)
**Exchange, ¼ c. (60 mL) serving:** 2 bread, 1½ fat
**Calories, ¼ c. (60 mL) serving:** 215

*From Kellogg's Test Kitchens.*

# Pizza Maria

| | | |
|---|---|---|
| 60 | Health Valley herb crackers | 60 |
| ½ c. | Health Valley Bellissimo pasta sauce | 125 mL |
| ½ t. | Health Valley Instead of Salt vegetable seasoning | 2 mL |
| ½ t. | Health Valley Instead of Salt all-purpose seasoning | 2 mL |
| 1½ oz. | cheddar cheese, cut into ⅛-in. (3-mm) cubes | 5 mL |
| | parsley sprigs for garnish | |

Place crackers on cookie sheet. Mix pasta sauce with seasonings, drop ¼ t. (1 mL) on each cracker, then top with 1 cheese cube. Bake at 400 °F (200 °C) for 5 minutes or until cheese melts. To serve, arrange on platter. Garnish with parsley sprigs. Serve at once.

**Yield:** 60 appetizer pizzas
**Exchange, 2 appetizer pizzas:** ½ bread
**Calories, 2 appetizer pizzas:** 30

*From Health Valley Foods.*

# Frosty Fruit Tidbits

| | | |
|---|---|---|
| 1⅓ c. | Cracklin' Oat Bran cereal | 340 mL |
| 1 medium | banana, cut in ¾-in. (18-mm) pieces | 1 medium |
| 1 c. | fresh strawberries, with larger berries cut in half | 250 mL |
| ½ c. | pineapple chunks | 125 mL |
| ¾ c. | lemon low-fat yogurt | 190 mL |

Using rolling pin or electric blender, crush cereal into fine crumbs. Place in small shallow bowl. Set aside. Spear fruit pieces with cocktail picks. Dip in yogurt. Coat bottom half of each fruit piece with crushed cereal. Place in pan lined with waxed paper. Freeze until firm. Serve frozen or slightly thawed.

**Yield:** 3½ dozen
**Exchange, 3 fruit pieces:** 1 fruit
**Calories, 3 fruit pieces:** 50

*From Kellogg's Test Kitchens.*

## Hot South Seas Relish

| | | |
|---|---|---|
| 1 c. | vinegar | 250 mL |
| 2 T. | chili powder | 30 mL |
| 1 t. | dry mustard | 5 mL |
| dash | salt | dash |
| 2 | green tomatoes, chopped | 2 |
| 1 | green pepper, chopped | 1 |
| 1 medium | onion, chopped | 1 medium |
| ½ t. | horseradish | 2 mL |

Heat vinegar, chili powder, mustard and salt in a saucepan. Bring to boil and cook for 10 minutes. Place vegetables in bowl, pour hot sauce over entire mixture. Marinate at room temperature until cool. Serve or refrigerate.

**Yield:** 2 c. (500 mL)
**Exchange, 1 T. (15 mL):** negligible
**Calories, 1 T. (15 mL):** negligible

## Corn Relish

An old standby with lots of fiber.

| | | |
|---|---|---|
| 1 c. | vinegar | 250 mL |
| ½ c. | granulated sugar replacement | 125 mL |
| 1 t. | dry mustard | 5 mL |
| 1 t. | salt | 5 mL |
| ¼ t. | turmeric | 1 mL |
| 2 c. | Green Giant whole kernel corn, drained | 500 mL |
| ¼ c. | cabbage, finely chopped | 60 mL |
| ½ c. | onion, chopped | 125 mL |
| ⅓ c. | red pepper, chopped | 90 mL |
| ¼ c. | green pepper, chopped | 60 mL |

Mix vinegar, sugar replacement, mustard, salt and turmeric in a saucepan; heat to the boiling point. Add vegetables. Boil until vegetables are tender. Pour into serving dish and refrigerate until completely chilled.

**Yield:** 3 c. (750 mL)
**Exchange, ⅓ c. (90 mL):** ½ bread
**Calories, ⅓ c. (90 mL):** 31

## Sweet & Sour Chutney

I like this chutney with fowl or pork. It has a spicy "bite" to it.

| | | |
|---|---|---|
| 3 c. | sour cherries | 750 mL |
| 3 c. | dark cherries | 750 mL |
| 2 c. | cider vinegar | 500 mL |
| 2 large | yellow onions, thinly sliced | 2 large |
| 1 c. | white raisins (sultanas) | 250 mL |
| ½ c. | fresh lemon juice | 125 mL |
| 3 T. | fresh ginger root, finely chopped | 45 mL |
| ½ t. | ground nutmeg | 2 mL |
| ½ t. | ground allspice | 2 mL |
| ¼ t. | ground red pepper | 1 mL |

Place cherries in a large enamel or glass saucepan. Crush slightly with a potato masher. Add remaining ingredients. Cook over medium heat until mixture boils. Reduce heat, simmer until mixture is very thick, about 2 to 4 hours. Stir occasionally to prevent sticking. Remove from heat; ladle into sterilized jars or freezer containers. Seal. Chutney keeps indefinitely in refrigerator or freezer.

*Note*: This recipe can be started on the burner and finished cooking in a slow oven (275 °F or 135 °C). Or you can cook the mixture in a slow cooker on LOW for 6 to 8 hours.

**Yield:** 4 c. (1 L)
**Exchange ¼ c. (60 mL):** 2 fruit
**Calories ¼ c. (60 mL):** 78

## Tomato-Avocado Relish

This relish has a nice fresh flavor.

| | | |
|---|---|---|
| 2 medium | tomatoes, chopped | 2 medium |
| 1 | ripe avocado | 1 |
| ½ t. | lemon juice | 2 mL |
| | salt and pepper | |

Place chopped tomatoes in a bowl. Peel avocado and chop into small pieces. Mix thoroughly with tomato. Stir in lemon juice. Place a plate or cover directly on top of tomato-avocado mixture. Weight the plate down into the mixture to be sure avocado is completely submersed in the liquid to prevent discoloration. Marinate for at least 6 hours. Drain thoroughly and chill. Before serving, sprinkle salt and pepper to please your taste.

**Yield:** 1 c. (250 mL)
**Exchange, 1 T. (15 mL):** ½ fat
**Calories, 1 T. (15 mL):** 26

# Salads

## Salade Nicoise

| | | |
|---|---|---|
| ½ c. | Dia-Mel red wine vinegar salad dressing | 125 mL |
| ½ c. | Dia-Mel Italian salad dressing | 125 mL |
| ½ t. | dried dill | 2 mL |
| ½ t. | oregano | 2 mL |
| dash | black pepper | dash |
| ½ | red or yellow onion, thinly sliced | ½ |
| 3 oz. | marinated artichoke hearts, drained | 90 g |
| 1 c. | fresh green beans, cut and trimmed or frozen French-style green beans, thawed and drained | 250 mL |
| 2 small | Boston lettuce, torn into bite-size pieces | 2 small |
| ½ | cucumber, sliced | ½ |
| 2 | tomatoes, cut in wedges | 2 |
| ½ c. | mushrooms, sliced | 125 mL |
| ¼ c. | radishes, sliced | 60 mL |
| ½ c. | red pepper, sliced in thin strips | 125 mL |
| 1 medium | potato, cooked and sliced | 1 medium |
| 7-oz. can | tuna, packed in water, rinsed | 200-g can |
| ¼ c. | pitted black olives, sliced | 60 mL |
| 1 | hard-cooked egg, chopped | 1 |

Combine salad dressing with dill, oregano and pepper. Marinate onion, artichoke hearts and green beans in dressing mixture for 2 to 3 hours. Before serving, combine the marinated vegetables and dressing with the remaining ingredients *except* the hard-cooked egg. Toss to mix well. Garnish with the chopped egg.

**Yield:** 4 servings
**Exchange 1 serving:** 2 lean meat, 3 vegetables
**Calories, 1 serving:** 180

*For you from The Estee Corporation.*

# Poinsettia Salad

| | | |
|---|---|---|
| 1 c. | Stone-Buhr brown rice, cooked | 250 mL |
| 7-oz. can | chunk-style tuna, drained | 200-g can |
| ½ c. | pecans, chopped | 125 mL |
| ⅓ c. | mayonnaise | 90 mL |
| 1 T. | lemon juice | 15 mL |
| ¼ t. | Tabasco sauce | 1 mL |
| 1 | canned whole pimiento | 1 |
| 6 | lettuce leaves | 6 |

Cook rice according to package directions. Rinse with cold water and drain well. Combine tuna, rice, pecans, mayonnaise, lemon juice and Tabasco sauce. Toss lightly until well mixed. Press into 6 individual moulds or use a ⅓-c. (90-mL) measure. Turn out each moulded salad onto a lettuce leaf. Cut pimiento into petal shapes and arrange on salads to resemble poinsettias.

**Yield:** 6 servings
**Exchange, 1 serving:** 2 bread, 1 high-fat meat, 2 fat
**Calories, 1 serving:** 335

*With the compliments of Arnold Foods Company, Inc.*

# Mushroom & Watercress Salad

This is a delightful new taste for most people.

| | | |
|---|---|---|
| 3 c. | snow-white mushrooms (medium size) | 750 mL |
| 2 T. | fresh lemon juice | 30 mL |
| 2 T. | white wine vinegar | 30 mL |
| 2 T. | olive oil | 30 mL |
| ⅓ c. | water | 90 mL |
| ½ t. | salt | 2 mL |
| ½ t. | dried tarragon, crushed | 2 mL |
| ¼ t. | ground basil | 1 mL |
| 1 c. | fresh watercress, chopped | 250 mL |

Clean and slice mushrooms; place in a medium bowl. Mix together the lemon juice, vinegar, oil, water, salt, tarragon and basil. Pour dressing over mushrooms, mixing carefully to completely coat the mushrooms. Marinate overnight in the refrigerator. Just before serving, drain extra dressing from mushrooms, add watercress and toss to completely mix. Divide among 8 chilled salad plates.

**Yield:** 8 servings
**Exchange, 1 serving:** ½ vegetable, 1 fat
**Calories, 1 serving:** 57

## Polynesian Cabbage Slaw

| 1 small | cabbage, shredded | 1 small |
| 8½-oz. can | pineapple chunks packed in juice | 230-g can |
| 1 | orange, diced | 1 |
| ¼ c. | green pepper, diced | 60 mL |
| ⅓ c. | Dia-Mel Thousand Island salad dressing | 90 mL |
| ⅓ c. | Dia-Mel French-style salad dressing | 90 mL |
| ⅓ c. | Dia-Mel catsup | 90 mL |

Drain pineapple chunks. In a large bowl, combine all ingredients and mix thoroughly. Chill before serving.
**Yield:** 6 servings
**Exchange, 1 serving:** 1 fruit, ½ vegetable
**Calories, 1 serving:** 55

*For you from The Estee Corporation.*

## Old-Time Carrot Slaw

A favorite slaw for your picnics.

| ⅓ c. | water | 90 mL |
| 2 T. | vegetable oil | 30 mL |
| 2 T. | white vinegar | 30 mL |
| 3 env. | aspartame sweetener | 3 env. |
| ½ t. | salt | 2 mL |
| dash | black pepper | dash |
| 3 c. | carrots, shredded | 750 mL |
| 8 | ripe olives, sliced | 8 |

Combine water, oil, vinegar, aspartame, salt and pepper. Stir to blend. Pour over carrots. Toss to completely coat. Garnish with olive slices. Cover tightly and chill thoroughly. Drain well before serving.
**Yield:** 6 servings
**Exchange, 1 serving:** 1 vegetable, 1 fat
**Calories, 1 serving:** 73

## Sweet-Sour Slaw

| 2 medium | red onions | 2 medium |
| 4 c. | cabbage, finely shredded | 1 mL |
| ½ c. | cider vinegar | 125 mL |
| 1 t. | dry mustard | 5 mL |
| 1 t. | salt | 5 mL |
| 1 t. | celery seeds | 5 mL |
| ¼ t. | cornstarch | 1 mL |

| ⅓ c. | granulated sugar replacement | 90 mL |
| 2 T. | vegetable oil | 30 mL |

Thinly slice the onions and separate them into rings. In a large bowl, alternate layers of the cabbage and onion rings. In a small saucepan, combine vinegar, mustard, salt, celery seeds and cornstarch. Stir to dissolve cornstarch. Cook over medium heat until mixture boils and is clear. Remove from heat, beat in sugar replacement and oil. Pour dressing over the cabbage. Cover tightly and refrigerate 8 hours or overnight, stirring occasionally. To serve, using a slotted spoon, lift salad out of the dressing.

**Yield:** 10 servings
**Exchange, 1 serving:** ½ fat
**Calories, 1 serving:** 25

## Apple-Cabbage Slaw

| ¼ c. | Dia-Mel creamy Italian salad dressing | 60 mL |
| ¼ t. | prepared mustard | 1 mL |
| dash | pepper | dash |
| 2 c. | cabbage, shredded | 500 mL |
| 1 c. | unpared apple, thinly sliced | 250 mL |

In a medium bowl, combine salad dressing, mustard and pepper. Add cabbage and apple and toss lightly. Serve immediately.

**Yield:** 4 servings
**Exchange, 1 serving:** 1½ vegetable
**Calories, 1 serving:** 35

*For you from The Estee Corporation.*

## Lemony Apple-Bran Salad

| ½ c. | lemon low-fat yogurt | 125 mL |
| 1 T. | fresh parsley, finely snipped | 15 mL |
| 2 c. | unpared red apples, cored and cubed | 500 mL |
| ½ c. | celery, thinly sliced | 125 mL |
| ½ c. | red grapes, halved and seeded | 125 mL |
| ½ c. | All-Bran or Bran Buds cereal | 125 mL |
| 6 | lettuce leaves | 6 |

Stir together yogurt, parsley, apples, celery and grapes. Cover and chill thoroughly. At serving time, stir in the cereal. Serve on lettuce leaves.

**Yield:** 6 servings
**Exchange, 1 serving:** 1 fruit, ½ bread
**Calories, 1 serving:** 70

*From Kellogg's Test Kitchens.*

## Hot Bean Salad

| | | |
|---|---|---|
| 2 c. | kidney beans, cooked and drained | 500 mL |
| 1 c. | celery, thinly sliced | 250 mL |
| ½ c. | sharp American cheese, diced | 125 mL |
| ¼ c. | sweet relish | 60 mL |
| ¼ c. | onions, coarsely chopped | 60 mL |
| ⅓ c. | low-cal mayonnaise | 90 mL |
| ½ t. | salt | 2 mL |
| ⅓ c. | wheat germ | 90 mL |

Combine beans, celery, cheese, relish, onions, mayonnaise and salt in a large bowl. Stir to mix thoroughly. Spoon into 8 custard cups or baking dishes. Sprinkle wheat germ on top. Bake at 450 °F (225 °C) for 10 minutes or until bubbly.
**Yield:** 8 servings
**Exchange, 1 serving:** ⅔ bread, 1 lean meat
**Calories, 1 serving:** 97

## Chilled Bean Salad

| | | |
|---|---|---|
| 15½-oz. can | no-salt-added green beans | 450-g can |
| 15½-oz. can | no-salt-added wax beans | 450-g can |
| 1 | red pepper, chopped | 1 |
| 12 | cherry tomatoes, cut in half | 2 |
| ½ t. | dried dill | 2 mL |
| ½ t. | dried basil | 2 mL |
| ¼ c. | Dia-Mel red wine vinegar salad dressing | 60 mL |

Drain green and wax beans and combine with the red pepper and tomatoes. Add dillweed and basil to salad dressing; stir to combine. Pour dressing over vegetables and toss gently. Chill for several hours or overnight.
**Yield:** 6 servings
**Exchange, 1 serving:** 1½ vegetable
**Calories, 1 serving:** 40

*For you from The Estee Corporation.*

## Vegetable-Bean Salad

| | | |
|---|---|---|
| 8-oz. can | Featherweight cut green beans, drained | 227-g can |
| 8-oz. can | Featherweight cut wax beans, drained | 227-g can |
| ½ c. | green or red pepper, chopped | 125 mL |
| ¼ c. | onion, sliced | 60 mL |
| ½ c. | Featherweight Italian dressing | 125 mL |
| 6 | lettuce leaves | 6 |

In a medium bowl, combine all ingredients except the lettuce. Cover and marinate overnight in the refrigerator. Serve on lettuce.

**Yield:** 6 servings

**Exchange 1 serving:** 1 vegetable

**Calories, 1 serving:** 31

*Based on a recipe from Featherweight Brand Foods.*

## Wilted Lettuce Salad

| | | |
|---|---|---|
| 2 T. | margarine | 30 mL |
| ¾ t. | paprika | 3 mL |
| ¼ t. | garlic salt | 1 mL |
| 1 T. | sesame seeds | 15 mL |
| 1 c. | All-Bran or Bran Buds cereal | 250 mL |
| 2 T. | Parmesan cheese, grated | 30 mL |
| 6 | bacon slices | 6 |
| 2 qts. | iceberg lettuce, torn into bite-size pieces | 2 L |
| 1 | tomato, chopped | 1 |
| ¼ c. | green onions, sliced | 60 mL |
| ½ t. | oregano | 2 mL |
| ¼ t. | pepper | 1 mL |
| ¼ c. | vinegar | 60 mL |
| 2 t. | sugar | 10 mL |

In a medium skillet, melt margarine over low heat. Stir in paprika, garlic salt and sesame seeds. Add cereal, stirring until well-coated. Cook, stirring constantly, 2 to 3 minutes or until cereal is crisp and lightly brown. Remove from heat. Add cheese, tossing lightly. Set aside.

Fry bacon until crisp. Drain, reserving 2 T. (30 mL) of the drippings. Crumble bacon into small pieces. Set aside. In a large bowl, toss lettuce with tomato, green onions, oregano and pepper. Set aside. Combine reserved bacon drippings, vinegar and sugar in a small saucepan. Bring to a boil. Pour over lettuce. Cover bowl about 1 minute. Portion salad into individual salad bowls. Sprinkle bacon and cereal mixture over each portion. Serve immediately.

**Yield:** 6 servings

**Exchange, 1 serving:** ½ bread, 2 vegetables, 2 fat

**Calories, 1 serving:** 175

*From Kellogg's Test Kitchens.*

## Minted Brown Rice Salad

| | | |
|---|---|---|
| 2½ c. | brown rice, cooked and hot | 625 mL |
| ⅓ c. | lemon juice | 90 mL |
| 2 T. | vegetable oil | 30 mL |
| ½ c. | fresh parsley, minced | 125 mL |
| ½ c. | fresh mint, minced | 125 mL |
| ¼ c. | green onions, thinly sliced | 60 mL |
| ½ c. | dates, finely chopped | 125 mL |
| ½ t. | salt | 2 mL |
| 2 | oranges | 2 |

Combine hot rice, lemon juice, oil, parsley, mint, onions, dates and salt in large bowl. Stir to completely blend. Cover and refrigerate until thoroughly chilled. Mound rice in a chilled, shallow serving dish. Peel oranges; slice crosswise. Decorate rice salad with the orange slices.
**Yield:** 6 servings
**Exchange, 1 serving:** 1 bread, 1 fruit, 1 fat
**Calories, 1 serving:** 155

## Tabbouleh

| | | |
|---|---|---|
| ½ c. | Stone-Buhr cracked wheat | 125 mL |
| 3 medium | fresh tomatoes, finely chopped | 3 medium |
| 1 c. | parsley, finely chopped | 250 mL |
| 1 c. | onion, finely chopped | 250 mL |
| ⅓ c. | fresh lemon juice | 90 mL |
| 2 t. | salt | 10 mL |
| 1 T. | vegetable oil | 15 mL |

Soak cracked wheat in cold water for about 10 minutes; drain. Wrap in cheese cloth and squeeze until dry. In large bowl, combine cracked wheat, tomatoes, parsley, onion, lemon juice and salt; toss lightly with a fork. Marinate at least half hour before serving. Just before serving, stir in the oil.
**Yield:** 8 servings
**Exchange, 1 serving:** ⅔ bread, ½ fat
**Calories, 1 serving:** 63
*With the compliments of Arnold Foods Company, Inc.*

## Tomatoes Vinaigrette

| | | |
|---|---|---|
| 2 large | tomatoes, unpeeled and thinly sliced | 2 large |
| 2 T. | water | 30 mL |
| 1 T. | vegetable oil | 15 mL |

| 1 T. | red wine vinegar | 15 mL |
| ¼ t. | salt | 1 mL |
| dash | dried basil | dash |
| dash | black pepper | dash |
| 2 T. | chive, chopped | 30 mL |

Arrange tomato slices on 4 serving plates. Combine water, oil, vinegar, salt, basil and pepper in a bowl or jar. Stir to completely blend. Sprinkle tomato slices with dressing. Garnish with chive.

**Yield:** 4 servings
**Exchange, 1 serving:** ½ vegetable, ½ fat
**Calories, 1 serving:** 42

## Mediterranean Eggplant Salad

A fast and interesting salad.

| ½ c. | long-grain brown rice | 125 mL |
| 1 medium | eggplant | 1 medium |
| 2 T. | vegetable oil | 30 mL |
| 1 t. | salt | 5 mL |
| 1 t. | ground cumin | 5 mL |
| 1 t. | ground cinnamon | 5 mL |
| 1 c. | celery, thinly sliced | 250 mL |
| ½ c. | green onion, thinly sliced | 125 mL |
| 2 | tomatoes | 2 |
| 8 large | lettuce leaves | 8 large |
| 8 oz. | lemon-flavored yogurt | 227 g |

Prepare the rice as directed on package. Wash the eggplant and remove stem. Cut into 1-in. (2.5-cm) cubes. Heat the oil in a large skillet. Add eggplant and cook, stirring, until eggplant starts to brown. Add a small amount of water, cover tightly and reduce heat. Uncover pan in short intervals and stir, adding extra water, if needed. Cook until eggplant is tender. Drain any excess liquid. Remove from pan and stir in the salt, cumin and cinnamon. Carefully stir in the rice. Cool to room temperature. Add celery and green onion. Place in bowl, cover and refrigerate until completely chilled, about 2 hours or overnight. Place the lettuce leaves on 8 chilled salad plates. Divide salad equally among plates. Cut tomatoes into eighths; garnish each salad with 2 tomato wedges. Top with equal amounts of yogurt.

**Yield:** 8 servings
**Exchange, 1 serving:** 1 bread, 1 fat
**Calories, 1 serving:** 109

## South-of-the-Border Salad Tray

This is a grand version of Pico de Gallo ("beak of the rooster") relish.

| | | |
|---|---|---|
| 2 medium | cucumbers | 2 medium |
| ½ c. | cider vinegar | 125 mL |
| 2 T. | vegetable oil | 30 mL |
| 1 t. | salt | 5 mL |
| 1 large | white onion | 1 large |
| 3 large | oranges | 3 large |
| 1 large | avocado | 1 large |
| 1 T. | lemon juice | 30 mL |
| ½ c. | cold water | 125 mL |
| | Bibb lettuce leaves | |
| ½ t. | red pepper | 2 mL |

With a vegetable parer, peel lengthwise strips from each cucumber to make alternating green and white stripes. Cut off the ends and thinly slice the cucumbers into rounds; place in a large bowl. Add vinegar, oil and salt. Mix and chill for at least 2 hours. (This can be made a day in advance.) To arrange salad, lift cucumbers from marinade, and save the marinade. Drain slightly. Peel onion and oranges and thinly slice lengthwise. Combine lemon juice and water in a small bowl. Peel and thinly slice the avocado; drop avocado slices into the lemon water to avoid discoloration. On a large platter or tray, arrange separate sections of cucumber, onion, orange and avocado slices. Garnish with lettuce leaves. Just before serving, combine reserved cucumber marinade with the red pepper. Pour over entire salad.

**Yield:** 12 servings
**Exchange, 1 serving:** ½ fruit, 1 fat
**Calories, 1 serving:** 67

## Creamy Potato Salad

A family favorite.

| | | |
|---|---|---|
| 2 lbs. | potatoes | 1 kg |
| 1½ t. | salt | 7 mL |
| ½ c. | green pepper, chopped | 125 mL |
| ¼ c. | onion, chopped | 60 mL |
| ¼ c. | wheat germ | 60 mL |
| ¼ c. | Dannon plain low-fat yogurt | 60 mL |
| ¼ c. | low-cal mayonnaise | 60 mL |
| 1 t. | lemon juice | 5 mL |

Put potatoes and 1 t. (5 mL) of the salt into a large saucepan; add water to cover completely. Bring to a boil, cover and reduce heat. Simmer for 20 to 25 minutes or until potatoes are just tender. *Do not overcook.* Drain potatoes and rinse with cold water; peel. Cut potatoes into 1-in. (2.5-cm) pieces. Combine remaining ingredients, pour over hot potatoes. Stir gently to completely blend. Cover tightly and refrigerate until chilled.

**Yield:** 6 servings
**Exchange, 1 serving:** 1½ bread
**Calories, 1 serving:** 128

## Plain Papaya Salad

| 2½ c. | papaya, diced | 625 mL |
|---|---|---|
| 2 c. | fresh pineapple, diced | 500 ml |
| 1 c. | celery, sliced | 250 mL |
| 2 T. | chive, chopped | 30 mL |
| ½ t. | salt | 2 mL |
| 6 large | lettuce leaves | 6 large |
| 6 T. | low-cal mayonnaise | 90 mL |

Combine papaya, pineapple, celery, chive and salt in a large bowl: fold to blend. Serve on a large lettuce leaf. Top with 1 T. (15 mL) mayonnaise, divided among the servings.

**Yield:** 6 servings
**Exchange, 1 serving:** 1 fruit, ½ fat
**Calories, 1 serving:** 69

## Cantaloupe-Strawberry Salad

A refreshing salad for summer.

| 2 | cantaloupes | 2 |
|---|---|---|
| 1 c. | fresh strawberries | 250 mL |
| 1 head | iceberg lettuce, cleaned | 1 head |
| 1 c. | Dannon lemon low-fat yogurt | 250 mL |

Cut cantaloupes into crosswise halves and remove seeds. Using a melon ball cutter, scoop the cantaloupes into balls. Tear lettuce into small pieces. Toss lettuce with yogurt in a large bowl. Arrange cantaloupe balls and strawberries in alternate circles on top of lettuce bed. Cover and chill thoroughly.

**Yield:** 8 servings
**Exchange, 1 serving:** 2 fruit
**Calories, 1 serving:** 58

## Autumn Fruit Bowl

In these fruits you have the colors of a maple tree in autumn.

| | | |
|---|---|---|
| 1 head | *romaine lettuce* | 1 head |
| 2 c. | *pineapple, cubed* | 500 mL |
| 1 | *grapefruit, segmented* | 1 |
| 1 | *apple, sliced and dipped in lemon juice* | 1 |
| 1 c. | *seedless red grapes* | 250 mL |
| 1 | *orange, segmented* | 1 |

Combine fruits in a large bowl. Cover tightly and refrigerate until thoroughly chilled. Line a large salad bowl with romaine lettuce leaves; spoon in the fruit. Serve immediately or chill until serving time.
**Yield:** 12 servings
**Exchange, 1 serving:** 1 fruit
**Calories, 1 serving:** 38

## Spinach-Orange-Chicken Salad

| | | |
|---|---|---|
| 4 oz. | *cooked chicken, cut in strips* | 125 g |
| 2 | *oranges, peeled and segmented* | 2 |
| ¼ c. | *red onion, thinly sliced* | 60 mL |
| 4 c. | *spinach, rinsed and torn into pieces* | 1 L |
| | *Orange Salad Dressing (recipe follows)* | |

In a salad bowl, toss together the first 4 ingredients. Add dressing and toss to coat.

### ORANGE SALAD DRESSING

| | | |
|---|---|---|
| 2 T. | *Mazola corn oil* | 30 mL |
| 2 T. | *orange juice* | 30 mL |
| 2 T. | *white wine vinegar* | 30 mL |
| ½ t. | *dry mustard* | 2 mL |
| ¼ t. | *ground ginger* | 1 mL |
| dash | *salt and pepper* | dash |

Into a small jar with a tight-fitting lid, measure all the ingredients. Cover and shake well. Chill. Shake before serving. Makes about ⅓ c. (90 mL).
**Yield:** 4 servings
**Exchange, 1 serving:** 2 lean meat, 1 fat
**Calories, 1 serving:** 160

*"A Diet for the Young at Heart" by Mazola.*

## Lemon Gazpacho Mould

| | | |
|---|---|---|
| 1 pkg. (2 env.) | Featherweight lemon gelatin | 1 pkg. (2 env.) |
| 1 t. | Featherweight instant bouillon, beef flavor | 5 mL |
| 1 c. | boiling water | 250 mL |
| 2½ c. | Featherweight tomato juice | 625 mL |
| 2 t. | red wine vinegar | 10 mL |
| 1 t. | Worcestershire sauce | 5 mL |
| ¼ t. | hot pepper sauce | 1 mL |
| 1 c. | unpared cucumber, chopped | 250 mL |
| ½ c. | celery, chopped | 125 mL |
| ½ c. | tomato, seeded and chopped | 125 mL |
| ¼ c. | green pepper, chopped | 60 mL |
| ¼ c. | onion, finely chopped | 60 mL |
| 2 6½-oz. cans | Featherweight tuna, drained and flaked | 2 190-g cans |

Empty both envelopes of gelatin into a bowl. Add bouillon and boiling water; stir until dissolved. Add tomato juice, vinegar, Worcestershire and pepper sauces; stir well. Refrigerate until thickened. Add cucumber, celery, tomato, green pepper, onion and tuna to the thickened gelatin; mix well. Turn mixture into a lightly oiled 5½- or 6-cup (1¼- or 1½-L) mould. Chill until firm. Unmould on a serving plate.
**Yield:** 6 servings
**Exchange, 1 serving:** 1½ lean meat, 1 vegetable
**Calories, 1 serving:** 101

*Based on a recipe from Featherweight Brand Foods.*

## Orange-Spinach Salad

| | | |
|---|---|---|
| ½ c. | Featherweight Russian dressing | 125 mL |
| ¼ c. | Featherweight orange marmalade | 60 mL |
| 10¼-oz. can | Featherweight mandarin oranges, drained | 300-g can |
| 12 oz. | spinach leaves, cleaned and torn in pieces | 360 g |
| ⅓ c. | unblanched almonds, sliced | 90 mL |

Mix dressing and marmalade in a bowl; add oranges. Cover and chill 1 hour. Combine spinach, almonds and fruit dressing in a salad bowl; toss gently.
**Yield:** 6 servings
**Exchange, 1 serving:** 1 fruit, 1 fat
**Calories, 1 serving:** 77

*Based on a recipe from Featherweight Brand Foods.*

## Classic Waldorf Salad

The always enjoyable fruit salad.

| | | |
|---|---|---|
| 4 c. | cold water | 1 L |
| ⅓ c. | lemon juice | 90 mL |
| 2 c. | apple, thinly sliced | 500 mL |
| 1 c. | celery, thinly sliced | 250 mL |
| ½ c. | walnuts, coarsely chopped | 125 mL |
| ¼ c. | low-cal mayonnaise | 60 mL |
| 2 T. | 2% milk | 30 mL |

Combine water and lemon juice. Drop apple slices into lemon water; soak for 5 to 10 minutes. Drain apple pieces and pat with paper towel until slightly dry. Combine apple, celery and walnuts in a bowl. In a cup, stir together the mayonnaise and milk; add to the apple mixture and toss to completely coat. Cover and chill thoroughly.
**Yield:** 6 servings
**Exchange, 1 serving:** 1 bread, 1½ fat
**Calories, 1 serving:** 135

## Post-Holiday Turkey Salad

| | | |
|---|---|---|
| 2 T. | vegetable oil | 30 mL |
| 2 T. | cider vinegar | 30 mL |
| ½ t. | curry powder | 2 mL |
| ½ t. | salt | 2 mL |
| dash | white pepper | dash |
| ½ t. | onion powder | 2 mL |
| 6-oz. pkg. | La Choy frozen pea pods, partially thawed | 180-g pkg. |
| 2 T. | pimientos, coarsely chopped | 30 mL |
| ½ c. | fresh mushrooms, sliced | 125 mL |
| 1½ c. | cooked turkey, cubed | 375 mL |
| 2 c. | iceberg lettuce, torn into pieces | 500 mL |
| ½ c. | celery, thinly sliced | 125 mL |

Shake together the oil, vinegar and seasonings in a jar with a tight-fitting lid. Dry pea pods between paper towels to remove excess moisture. In medium bowl, combine pea pods, pimientos, mushrooms, and turkey. Add dressing; toss lightly. Cover; chill for about 1 hour, tossing once or twice. In a salad bowl, toss lightly the pea pod mixture with lettuce and celery.
**Yield:** 4 servings
**Exchange, 1 serving:** 2 lean meat, ½ fat
**Calories, 1 serving:** 142

*Adapted from recipes from La Choy Food Products.*

# Gala Salad

| | | |
|---|---|---|
| 14-oz. can | La Choy bean sprouts, rinsed and drained | 420-g can |
| 1 c. | fresh mushrooms, thinly sliced | 250 mL |
| 3 T. | lemon juice | 45 mL |
| 1 T. | sesame oil | 15 mL |
| 1 t. | liquid fructose | 5 mL |
| 1 t. | salt | 5 mL |
| ¼ t. | onion powder | 1 mL |
| 2 c. | cooked chicken, diced | 500 mL |
| 3 T. | pimiento, chopped | 45 mL |
| 1 T. | sesame seeds, toasted | 15 mL |

Cover bean sprouts with ice water; let stand for 30 minutes. Drain well. Place bean sprouts and mushrooms in mixing bowl. In another bowl, blend together lemon juice, oil, liquid fructose, salt and onion powder. Add to vegetables; toss lightly. Chill. Just before serving, add chicken, pimiento and sesame seeds; toss lightly. Serve on crips salad greens.
**Yield:** 4 servings
**Exchange, 1 serving:** 2 lean meat
**Calories, 1 serving:** 120

*Adapted from a La Choy Food Products recipe.*

# Soy Chicken Salad

A lovely salad to serve on a hot July day.

| | | |
|---|---|---|
| 2 c. | chicken, cooked and shredded | 500 mL |
| ½ c. | cucumber, sliced | 125 mL |
| ½ c. | alfalfa sprouts | 125 mL |
| 1 | egg, hard-cooked and chopped | 1 |
| 2 T. | lemon juice | 30 mL |
| 1 T. | vegetable oil | 15 mL |
| 2 t. | water | 10 mL |
| 2 t. | soy sauce | 10 mL |
| ½ t. | Dijon-style mustard | 2 mL |
| dash | black pepper | dash |

Combine chicken, cucumber, sprouts and egg in a medium bowl. Cover tightly and refrigerate until serving time. To make the dressing, blend remaining ingredients. Just before serving, pour dressing over salad. Toss to completely coat the salad.
**Yield:** 3 c. (750 mL)
**Exchange, 1 c. (250 mL):** 2 lean meat, ½ vegetable
**Calories, 1 c. (250 mL):** 123

# Vegetable Aspic

| | | |
|---|---|---|
| 2 env. | unflavored gelatin | 2 env. |
| ¼ c. | cold water | 60 mL |
| 3½ c. | fresh tomato, cut into wedges | 875 mL |
| ½ c. | celery leaves, finely chopped | 125 mL |
| 1 c. | white onion, chopped | 250 mL |
| 3 T. | fresh parsley, minced | 45 mL |
| 1 | bay leaf | 1 |
| 1 t. | salt | 5 mL |
| ¼ t. | pepper | 1 mL |
| 1 c. | celery, sliced | 250 mL |
| 1 c. | cabbage, shredded | 250 mL |

Soften gelatin in cold water; set aside. Combine tomato wedges, celery leaves, onions, parsley, bay leaf, salt and pepper in a saucepan. Cook and stir over medium heat for 15 minutes. Pour small amount of tomato mixture into softened gelatin, then add to the saucepan. Cook and stir until gelatin is completely dissolved. Remove from heat. Discard bay leaf. Cool in refrigerator until mixture starts to thicken. Fold in celery and cabbage. Pour into slightly oiled mould or serving dish. Refrigerate until completely set.

**Yield:** 6 servings
**Exchange, 1 serving:** 1 vegetable
**Calories, 1 serving:** 22

# Green Bean Salad

A favorite for many people. Fast and easy with a nice tang.

| | | |
|---|---|---|
| 3 c. | green beans, cooked | 750 mL |
| 1 small | red onion, finely chopped | 1 small |
| ½ c. | radishes, sliced | 125 mL |
| ½ c. | low-cal french dressing | 125 mL |
| 1½ c. | lettuce, finely shredded | 375 mL |

Combine beans, onions and radishes with the dressing. Divide shredded lettuce equally among 6 chilled serving dishes. With a slotted spoon, scoop equal amounts of bean salad onto the lettuce bed.

**Yield:** 6 servings
**Exchange, 1 serving:** 1 vegetable, ¼ fat
**Calories, 1 serving:** 35

# Quick Bulgur Salad

A salad that also can be used as a stuffing for a pita sandwich.

| | | |
|---|---|---|
| ⅓ c. | fresh lemon juice | 90 mL |
| 2 t. | fresh lemon peel, finely chopped | 10 mL |
| 2 T. | olive oil | 30 mL |
| 2 t. | salt | 10 mL |
| ¼ t. | black pepper, freshly ground | 1 mL |
| 1 c. | bulgur wheat | 250 mL |
| 1 c. | boiling water | 250 mL |
| ½ c. | fresh parsley, chopped | 125 mL |
| ½ c. | red onion, finely chopped | 125 mL |
| 2 c. | tomatoes, chopped | 500 mL |

Combine lemon juice, lemon peel, oil, salt and pepper in a shaker bottle. Place bulgur in ovenproof bowl, add boiling water. Stir to blend. Cover tightly, allow to stand for 10 to 15 minutes or until all the water is absorbed. Toss with 2 forks to separate grains. Shake dressing and pour over bulgur; toss to thoroughly mix. Add remaining ingredients; toss again. Serve at room temperature.

**Yield:** 3 c. (750 mL)
**Exchange, ½ c. (125 mL):** 1 bread, 1 fat
**Calories, ½ c. (125 mL):** 125

# Marinated Potato Salad

| | | |
|---|---|---|
| ¼ c. | Mazola corn oil | 60 mL |
| ¼ c. | green onion, thinly sliced | 60 mL |
| 2 T. | white wine vinegar | 30 mL |
| 2 T. | dry white wine | 30 mL |
| 1 T. | parsley, chopped | 15 mL |
| ½ t. | dried dill | 2 mL |
| ¼ t. | salt | 1 mL |
| ¼ t. | pepper | 1 mL |
| 2 lb. | red potatoes, cooked, sliced ¼-in. (6-mm) thick | 1 kg |

In a large bowl, stir together the first 8 ingredients. Add potatoes. Gently toss to coat potatoes. Cover; chill for several hours, tossing occasionally. If desired, salad may be served warm.

**Yield:** 6 servings
**Exchange, 1 serving:** 1½ bread, 2 fat
**Calories, 1 serving:** 200

*"A Diet for the Young at Heart" by Mazola.*

# Vegetables

## Cauliflower au Gratin

| | | |
|---|---|---|
| 10-oz. pkg. | cauliflower, thawed | 280-g pkg. |

**Sauce**

| | | |
|---|---|---|
| 1 T. | butter | 15 mL |
| 1 T. | Stone-Buhr all purpose flour | 15 mL |
| 1/4 t. | salt | 1 mL |
| dash | pepper | dash |
| 1 t. | dry mustard | 5 mL |
| 3/4 c. | skim milk | 190 mL |
| 1/2 c. | cheddar cheese, grated | 125 mL |

**Topping**

| | | |
|---|---|---|
| 1/4 c. | Stone-Buhr wheat germ | 60 mL |
| 1/4 c. | Stone-Buhr bran flakes | 60 mL |
| 2 t. | butter, melted | 10 mL |
| 1/4 t. | dried sage | 1 mL |
| dash | dry mustard | dash |
| dash | salt | dash |

Spread cauliflower in bottom of ungreased 1-qt. (1-L) casserole. To prepare cheese sauce, melt butter in a saucepan and blend in flour and seasonings; stir until smooth. Remove from heat and stir in milk. Heat to boiling, stirring constantly. Add grated cheese and stir until melted and mixture is thickened. Pour sauce over cauliflower.

Combine the topping ingredients and sprinkle over the sauce. Bake uncovered at 325 °F (165 °C) for 15 minutes or until vegetable is heated through and crispy-tender.

**Microwave:** Combine ingredients as above. Cook at MEDIUM for 3 minutes; turn and cook 2 minutes longer.

**Yield:** 5 servings
**Exchange, 1 serving:** 2 vegetable, 1 fat
**Calories, 1 serving:** 88

*With the compliments of Arnold Foods Company, Inc.*

## Cauliflower Crunch

| | | |
|---|---|---|
| ½ c. | Kretschmer regular wheat germ | 125 mL |
| ¼ c. | Parmesan cheese, grated | 60 mL |
| 1 t. | paprika | 5 mL |
| ½ t. | dried tarragon, crushed | 2 mL |
| ½ t. | salt | 2 mL |
| dash | pepper | dash |
| ¼ c. | margarine, melted | 60 mL |
| 1 head | cauliflower, cut into florets | 1 head |

Combine wheat germ, cheese, paprika, tarragon, salt and pepper in a plastic bag. Toss together the melted margarine and cauliflower in a bowl until coated. Shake cauliflower, a third at a time, with crumb mixture in plastic bag until coated. Place on 15½ × 10½ × 1-in. (39 × 25 × 3-cm) jelly roll pan. Bake at 375 °F (190 °C) for 10 to 12 minutes until crisp-tender.

**Yield:** 6 servings
**Exchange, 1 serving:** 1 vegetable, ½ bread, 1½ fat
**Calories, 1 serving:** 123

   With the courtesy of Kretschmer Wheat Germ/International Multifoods.


## Baked Red Onions

So easy to prepare, this vegetable dish features red onions—try it!

| | | |
|---|---|---|
| 2 large | red onions | 2 large |
| 1 T. | red wine vinegar | 15 mL |
| 3 T. | water | 45 mL |
| 2 t. | granulated sugar replacement | 10 mL |
| ½ t. | salt | 2 mL |
| ¼ t. | ground sage | 1 mL |
| ¼ t. | dry mustard | 1 mL |
| 2 T. | margarine | 30 mL |

Peel and cut onions in half crosswise. Place side by side, cut side up, in a shallow 8-in. (20-cm) baking pan. In a small bowl, blend together the vinegar, water, sugar replacement, salt, sage and mustard. Pour over onion halves. Cover tightly. Bake at 350 °F (175 °C) for 50 to 60 minutes or until onions are tender.

**Microwave:** Reduce water to 2 T. (30 mL). Cook on HIGH for 5 to 10 minutes, turning dish every 3 minutes.

**Yield:** 4 servings
**Exchange, 1 serving:** 1 vegetable
**Calories, 1 serving:** 30

## Sautéed Oriental Beans

| | | |
|---|---|---|
| 2 t. | low-cal margarine | 10 mL |
| ¼ c. | white onion, chopped | 60 mL |
| 2 c. | bean sprouts | 500 mL |
| 1 T. | soy sauce | 15 mL |

Melt margarine in a nonstick saucepan. Over medium heat, lightly sauté onions until translucent. Add bean sprouts. Reduce heat, cover and cook 3 minutes. Toss with soy sauce. Serve immediately.
**Yield:** 4 servings
**Exchange, 1 serving:** 1 vegetable
**Calories, 1 serving:** 28

## Stir-Fried Broccoli

| | | |
|---|---|---|
| 2 T. | Mazola corn oil | 30 mL |
| 1 lb. | broccoli, cut in florets, and stems sliced | 500 g |
| 1¼ c. | mushrooms | 310 mL |
| 1 clove | garlic, minced | 1 clove |
| ¼ t. | dried thyme | 1 mL |
| ¼ t. | black pepper | 1 mL |

In a large skillet, heat oil over medium high heat. Add remaining ingredients. Stir-fry 5 to 8 minutes or until crisp-tender.
**Yield:** 4 servings
**Exchange, 1 serving:** 2 vegetable, 1 fat
**Calories, 1 serving:** 110

*"A Diet for the Young at Heart" by Mazola.*

## Brussels Sprouts in Yogurt Sauce

| | | |
|---|---|---|
| 2 lbs. | brussels sprouts | 1 kg |
| 8 oz. | Dannon plain low-fat yogurt | 227 g |
| 2 T. | cream of wheat cereal | 30 mL |
| | freshly ground pepper | |
| | salt to taste | |

Trim any wilted leaves or woody stem sections from the brussels sprouts. Put brussels sprouts in a steamer over boiling water and cook until just crisp-tender (*do not overcook*). Combine yogurt and cereal in a small saucepan. Cook and stir over low heat until mixture thickens. Pour sauce over hot brussels sprouts. Sprinkle with pepper and salt.
**Yield:** 8 servings
**Exchange, 1 serving:** 1 vegetable, ½ nonfat milk
**Calories, 1 serving:** 61

## Brussels Sprouts with Cream Sauce

| | | |
|---|---|---|
| 3 c. | *fresh brussels sprouts* | *750 mL* |
| 2 T. | *margarine* | *30 mL* |
| 2 T. | *Stone-Buhr dark rye flour* | *30 mL* |
| ¼ t. | *salt* | *1 mL* |
| 1 c. | *skim milk* | *250 mL* |

Trim off the stem and discolored leaves from the brussels sprouts; cook in salted water for 15 minutes. Drain and cover with boiling salted water. Cook, uncovered, just until tender, about 15 minutes. Meanwhile, to make the sauce, melt the margarine in a pan. Add the flour and salt and mix thoroughly. Stir in the milk and bring to a boil, stirring occasionally. Set aside over low heat until brussels sprouts are cooked. Drain brussels sprouts and place in a heated serving bowl. Pour sauce over vegetables and serve.

**Yield:** 6 servings
**Exchange, 1 serving:** 1 vegetable, 1 fat
**Calories, 1 serving:** 62

*With the compliments of Arnold Foods Company, Inc.*

## Broccoli & Pasta with Cheese

A side dish that includes a bread, vegetable and fat exchange.

| | | |
|---|---|---|
| 1¼ lbs. | *fresh broccoli* | *625 g* |
| 2 T. | *salt* | *30 mL* |
| ½ lb. | *small shell pasta* | *250 g* |
| 16 | *cherry tomatoes, halved* | *16* |
| 1 clove | *garlic, minced* | *1 clove* |
| ¼ c. | *Parmesan cheese, grated* | *60 mL* |

Cut florets from broccoli head and slice stems crosswise into ½-in. (13-mm) pieces. In a large saucepan, heat 2 qts. (2 L) water to the boiling point. Add broccoli and 1 T. (15 mL) of the salt. Cook 4 to 5 minutes or until crisp-tender. Drain in strainer or colander. In the same pan, bring 3 qts. (3 L) water to the boiling point. Add pasta and 1 T. (15 mL) salt to water; cook until pasta is *al dente* ("firm to the teeth"). Remove from heat but do not drain. Add tomato halves and garlic to hot pasta and water. Cover and allow to rest for 5 minutes. Add broccoli and reheat slightly. Drain in strainer or colander. While in strainer, sprinkle mixture with half the cheese, toss lightly and repeat with remaining cheese. Pour into hot serving bowl.

**Yield:** 8 servings
**Exchange, 1 serving:** 1 bread, 1 vegetable, 1 fat
**Calories, 1 serving:** 146

## Crumb-Topped Zucchini & Tomatoes

| | | |
|---|---|---|
| ¾ c. | Kellogg's bran flakes cereal | 190 mL |
| 2 t. | margarine | 10 mL |
| ½ t. | lemon peel, grated | 2 mL |
| 3 c. | zucchini, cut in ¼-in. (6-mm) slices | 750 mL |
| 2 T. | margarine | 30 mL |
| ¼ t. | salt | 1 mL |
| dash | pepper | dash |
| 1 T. | lemon juice | 15 mL |
| 3 | tomatoes, cut in wedges | 3 |

Crush cereal to make crumbs. Melt the 2 t. (10 mL) margarine in small skillet. Stir in cereal crumbs. Cook over low heat, stirring constantly, until lightly browned. Remove from heat. Stir in lemon peel. Set aside for topping.

In large skillet, cook zucchini in the 2 T. (30 mL) margarine until almost tender, stirring frequently. Sprinkle with salt and pepper. Stir in lemon juice and tomato wedges. Continue cooking until tomatoes are heated. Spoon vegetable mixture into serving bowl. Top with cereal mixture. Serve immediately.

**Yield:** 6 servings
**Exchange, 1 serving:** 2 vegetables, 1 fat
**Calories, 1 serving:** 85

*From Kellogg's Test Kitchens.*


## Peppers & Tomatoes

| | | |
|---|---|---|
| 1 medium | onion, chopped | 1 medium |
| 2 cloves | garlic, minced | 2 cloves |
| 1 T. | vegetable oil | 15 mL |
| 1 c. | green pepper, sliced into sticks | 250 mL |
| ½ c. | sweet red pepper, cut into chunks | 125 mL |
| 5 | tomatoes, cored and quartered | 5 |
| 1 | bay leaf | 1 |
| 2 T. | fresh parsley, chopped | 30 mL |

In a heavy pan, sauté onion and garlic in the oil until golden brown. Add peppers. Reduce heat, cover and cook 5 minutes. Add tomatoes and bay leaf. Cover and cook for 5 minutes longer. Pour into serving dish. Season with salt and pepper. Garnish with parsley and serve warm.

**Yield:** 6 servings
**Exchange, 1 serving:** 1 vegetable, ½ fat
**Calories, 1 serving:** 42

# Zucchini Patties

| ⅓ c. | Kretschmer regular wheat germ | 90 mL |
| ⅓ c. | all-purpose flour | 90 mL |
| ¼ c. | Parmesan cheese, grated | 60 mL |
| ¼ t. | baking powder | 1 mL |
| ¼ t. | oregano, crushed | 1 mL |
| dash | salt | dash |
| 2 c. | zucchini (about 2 medium), shredded | 500 mL |
| 2 | eggs, slightly beaten | 2 |

Combine wheat germ, flour, cheese, baking powder, oregano and salt in a bowl. Stir well to blend. Add zucchini and eggs. Stir just to blend. Preheat griddle to 350 °F (175 °C). It is ready when drops of water skitter on the surface. Grease hot griddle for the first patties. Drop batter by spoonfuls onto griddle, spreading to flatten slightly. Bake until golden brown, about 3 to 4 minutes. Turn and bake other side about 3 to 4 minutes. Continue making patties. Serve with favorite main dish, if desired.

**Yield:** 12 small patties
**Exchange, 2 patties:** 2 vegetables, ½ fat
**Calories, 2 patties:** 80

*With the courtesy of Kretschmer Wheat Germ/International Multifoods.*

# Creamed Beets

The lovely color invites you to any table.

| 2 T. | butter | 30 mL |
| 3 T. | all-purpose flour | 45 mL |
| 1 c. | water | 250 mL |
| 2 T. | lemon juice | 30 mL |
| 1 small | bay leaf | 1 small |
| 2 c. | small beets, cooked and diced | 500 mL |
| 1 env. | aspartame sweetener | 1 env. |
| | salt to taste | |

Melt butter in a heavy or nonstick fry pan. Add flour and stir over low heat for 1 minute. Mix water with lemon juice; slowly add to pan, stirring constantly, to blend into a smooth mixture. Add bay leaf. Cook until thickened. Add beets and cook until hot. Remove from heat and discard bay leaf. Add aspartame sweetener and salt.

**Yield:** 6 servings
**Exchange, 1 serving:** 1 vegetable, 1 fat
**Calories, 1 serving:** 76

## Spicy Cabbage

| 3 c. | cabbage, shredded | 750 mL |
| 1 t. | mixed pickling spices | 5 mL |
| 2 cloves | garlic, minced | 2 cloves |
| ¼ c. | wine vinegar | 60 mL |
| 1 t. | salt | 5 mL |
| ¼ t. | red pepper | 1 mL |

Combine all ingredients in large saucepan. Cover, cook until cabbage is crisp-tender. Drain.

**Yield:** 4 servings
**Exchange, 1 serving:** ½ vegetable
**Calories, 1 serving:** 11

## Sweet Cabbage

Don't snub this dish until you try it. It's good!

| ¼ c. | water | 60 mL |
| 6 c. | cabbage, finely shredded | ½ L |
| 2 T. | cider vinegar | 30 mL |
| ½ t. | salt | 2 mL |
| 2 medium | apples, unpeeled and finely sliced | 2 medium |
| ½ t. | granulated sugar replacement | 2 mL |

In a large saucepan, bring water to boil, add cabbage, vinegar and salt. Stir to mix. Cover and cook over medium heat for 20 to 25 minutes or until cabbage is tender. Add apple slices and sugar replacement to cabbage. Cook for 5 minutes longer. Serve hot.

**Microwave:** Place cabbage in 2-qt. (2-L) casserole. Add 2 T. (30 mL) water, vinegar and salt. Stir to mix. Cover tightly. Cook on HIGH for 8 to 10 minutes, turning dish once. Add apples and sugar replacement. Cover and cook for 3 minutes.

**Yield:** 5 c. (1¼ L)
**Exchange, 1 c. (250 mL):** 1 fruit or 1½ vegetable
**Calories, 1 c. (250 mL):** 40

## Sweet & Sour Sauerkraut

I tasted sauerkraut prepared this way at a local church fair. Thought you might like to try it.

| | | |
|---|---|---|
| 3 c. | homemade or canned sauerkraut, drained | 750 mL |
| 1 c. | crushed pineapple in its juice | 250 mL |
| 1 large | white onion | 1 large |
| 1 t. | pepper | 5 mL |

Combine ingredients in saucepan. Cover and cook over medium heat until onion is tender and most of the liquid has evaporated. Serve hot.
**Yield:** 6 servings
**Exchange, 1 serving:** 1 fruit
**Calories, 1 serving:** 43

## Light & Lively Cabbage Dish

This is microwave-fast to prepare and looks so pretty at the table.

| | | |
|---|---|---|
| 1 c. | cabbage, finely shredded | 250 mL |
| 1 c. | cauliflower, chopped | 250 mL |
| 1 medium | carrot, thinly sliced | 1 medium |
| 2 T. | water | 30 mL |
| 2 t. | butter | 10 mL |
| 1 t. | salt | 5 mL |
| ½ t. | white pepper | 2 mL |

Combine cabbage, cauliflower, carrot and water in a serving bowl. Cover tightly with plastic wrap. Microwave on HIGH for 8 minutes, turning dish once. Drain any excess water. Add butter, salt and white pepper. Stir to mix.
**Yield:** 2 c. (500 mL)
**Exchange, ½ c. (125 mL):** ½ vegetable, ½ fat
**Calories, ½ c. (125 mL):** 37

## Corn on the Grill

I have grilled corn on the cob many times, but this is my favorite version. This recipe is suggested for just one ear of corn. Repeat this procedure for each cob you plan to serve.

| | | |
|---|---|---|
| 5-in.-long ear | corn, unhusked | 12-cm-long ear |
| 1 t. | butter, melted | 5 mL |
| ½ t. | soy sauce | 2 mL |
| | salt and pepper to taste | |

Carefully, turn back husk from corn. Remove and discard corn silk. Wash corn, allowing husk to get wet. Add butter to soy sauce and brush corn with the mixture, then rewrap husk around corn. Wrap cob in aluminum foil. Grill 6 in. (15 cm) over heated coals for 10 to 12 minutes. Remove foil and husk. Season with salt and pepper.

**Yield:** 1 serving
**Exchange, 1 serving:** 3 vegetable, 1 fat
**Calories, 1 serving:** 115

## Corn Custard

Fresh or frozen corn can be substituted for canned corn in this no-fuss corn casserole.

| | | |
|---|---|---|
| 2 T. | all-purpose flour | 30 mL |
| ½ t. | salt | 2 mL |
| dash | pepper | dash |
| 16-oz. can | whole kernel corn, drained | 456-g can |
| 1 | egg | 1 |
| ¾ c. | nonfat milk | 190 mL |
| 1 T. | margarine, melted | 15 mL |
| ⅓ c. | All-Bran cereal | 90 mL |

Stir together the flour, salt and pepper. Toss with corn. In another bowl, beat egg slightly. Combine with milk and margarine and stir into corn mixture. Pour into round 1-qt. (1-L) casserole. Sprinkle with cereal. Bake at 325 °F (165 °C) for about 50 minutes or until knife inserted near middle comes out clean.

**Yield:** 4 servings
**Exchange, 1 serving:** 1 bread, 2 vegetable, 1 fat
**Calories, 1 serving:** 170

*From Kellogg's Test Kitchens.*

## Cheesy Dilled Carrots

| 16-oz. can | Featherweight sliced carrots, drained | 460-g can |
| ½ t. | dried dill | 2 mL |
| 5 T. | Featherweight cheddar cheese, shredded | 75 mL |

Toss together the carrots and dill in a 2-cup (500-mL) casserole. Top with cheese. Bake at 350 °F (175 °C) for 12 to 15 minutes or until cheese melts and carrots are piping hot.

**Yield:** 4 servings
**Exchange, 1 serving:** 1 vegetable, 1 fat
**Calories, 1 serving:** 71

*Based on a recipe from Featherweight Brand Foods.*

## Colorful Carrot & Green Bean Ring

A pretty vegetable dish—like this one—pleases both the eye and the appetite.

| 2 large | carrots, peeled | 2 large |
| 1 c. | green beans, canned | 250 mL |
| 1 large | snow-white mushroom, chopped | 1 large |
| | salt and black pepper to taste | |

Cut carrots into large pieces and finely grate them. Ring a plate or flat soup bowl with the grated carrots. Add a few drops of water. Cover tightly with plastic wrap. Microwave on HIGH for 4 minutes. Meanwhile, chop the green beans and mushroom but keep them separated. Uncover carrots and place green beans in the central section of the ring. Top the very middle with the chopped mushroom. Cover tightly with plastic. Microwave on MEDIUM for 4 minutes. Season with salt and pepper.

**Yield:** 4 servings
**Exchange, 1 serving:** 1 vegetable
**Calories, 1 serving:** 25

## Asparagus to Perfection

I love asparagus—I just wish it weren't so expensive.

| | | |
|---|---|---|
| 1 lb. | *fresh asparagus* | 500 g |
| ½ lb. | *fresh mushrooms* | 250 g |
| 1 T. | *butter* | 15 mL |
| ½ t. | *salt* | 2 mL |
| 1 t. | *La Choy soy sauce* | 5 mL |
| ½ c. | *water* | 125 mL |
| ½ t. | *cornstarch* | 2 mL |

Wash asparagus and break off and discard the woody parts. Place spears on cutting board and slice diagonally into thin slices. Clean and slice mushrooms. Melt butter in a skillet; add asparagus and mushrooms. Stir to coat. Add salt and soy sauce; cook, stirring, for 4 minutes. Combine water and cornstarch in bowl or shaker jar. Blend completely. Add to asparagus. Cook until cornstarch mixture clears and slightly thickens.

**Yield:** 4 servings
**Exchange, 1 serving:** 1 vegetable, 1 fat
**Calories, 1 serving:** 65

## Baked Spinach

I like to serve this for company. It can be made up in advance and popped into the oven at the last minute.

| | | |
|---|---|---|
| 2 lbs. | *fresh spinach* | 1 kg |
| 2 T. | *salad oil* | 30 mL |
| 2 c. | *onion, chopped* | 500 mL |
| 1 clove | *garlic, minced* | 1 clove |
| 2 | *eggs, beaten* | 2 |
| ½ c. | *Parmesan cheese, grated* | 125 mL |

Thoroughly wash and clean spinach. Drain. In a large fry pan, heat oil. Add onion and garlic, cook and stir until onion is transparent but not browned. Add spinach; cover tightly. Reduce heat and cook until spinach wilts. Pour spinach mixture into a greased casserole. In a bowl, combine the eggs with the cheese. Pour over top of spinach. (You may now refrigerate spinach until ready to bake.) Bake, uncovered, at 375 °F (190 °C) for about 15 minutes.

**Yield:** 8 servings
**Exchange, 1 serving:** 1 vegetable, ½ lean meat, 1 fat
**Calories, 1 serving:** 102

# Creamed Spinach

An Italian touch for spinach.

| | | |
|---|---|---|
| 1 T. | butter | 15 mL |
| 1 c. | onion, finely chopped | 250 mL |
| 2 cloves | garlic, minced | 2 cloves |
| 2 T. | all-purpose flour | 30 mL |
| ¾ c. | skim milk | 190 mL |
| ¼ t. | ground oregano | 1 mL |
| | salt and pepper to taste | |
| 2 lbs. | fresh spinach, cleaned and cooked | 1 kg |

Melt butter in a skillet. Add onion and garlic; cook over medium heat until onion is soft. Stir in flour; blend well. Remove pan from heat, slowly stir in milk, oregano, salt and pepper. Return to heat and cook 1 minute. Remove skillet from heat; add spinach and fold to mix. Turn into a well-greased baking dish. Bake uncovered at 375 °F (190 °C) for 12 to 15 minutes.

**Yield:** 6 servings
**Exchange, 1 serving:** 2 vegetable, ½ fat
**Calories, 1 serving:** 72

# Heavenly Eggplant Slices

A bouquet of spicy flavors for eggplant.

| | | |
|---|---|---|
| 1 large | eggplant | 1 large |
| 2 T. | vegetable oil | 30 mL |
| 3 | tomatoes, cored and cubed | 3 |
| 1 medium | yellow onion, finely chopped | 1 medium |
| 1 t. | granulated sugar replacement | 5 mL |
| 1 t. | ginger root, finely chopped | 5 mL |
| ¼ t. | ground ginger | 1 mL |
| ¼ t. | salt | 1 mL |
| dash | pepper | dash |
| 3 T. | fresh parsley, chopped | 45 mL |

Slice unpeeled eggplant in 1-in. (2.5-cm) slices. Brush oil on both sides of slices. Arrange in single layer in a baking dish. Place tomatoes in blender; blend to a purée. In a large saucepan, combine tomato pureé, onion, sugar replacement, ginger root, ground ginger, salt and pepper. Cook and stir over medium heat until onions are translucent. Pour sauce over eggplant slices. Bake at 400 °F (200 °C) for 20 to 30 minutes or until eggplant is tender. Garnish with parsley.

**Yield:** 6 servings
**Exchange, 1 serving:** ½ vegetable, 1 fat
**Calories, 1 serving:** 55

## Celery with Pearl Onions

| | | |
|---|---|---|
| 1 qt. | celery, thickly sliced | 1 L |
| 1 c. | pearl onions, peeled | 250 mL |
| 3 T. | dry sherry | 45 mL |
| 2 T. | water | 30 mL |
| ¼ t. | ground or grated nutmeg | 1 mL |
| ½ t. | salt | 2 mL |
| ¼ t. | black pepper | 1 mL |
| 1 T. | butter | 15 mL |

Combine celery and onions in large microwave bowl. Mix together the sherry, water and nutmeg. Pour over vegetables. Microwave on HIGH for 7 minutes, turning bowl once. Drain any excess liquid. Mix in salt, pepper and butter. Serve hot.

**Yield:** 6 servings
**Exchange, 1 serving:** 1 vegetable, ½ fat
**Calories, 1 serving:** 40

## A Side Dish of Mushrooms

Serve mushrooms often as a major vegetable. Here is a very quick way to prepare an impressive dish of mushrooms.

| | | |
|---|---|---|
| 1 lb. | fresh mushrooms | 500 g |
| 2 T. | water | 30 mL |
| 1 T. | soy sauce | 15 mL |
| | black pepper to taste (optional) | |

Clean and slice mushrooms. Heat a nonstick skillet. Add water and soy sauce. Heat slightly and add mushrooms. Cook and stir until mushrooms are tender. Season with pepper, if desired. Serve hot.

**Yield:** 4 servings
**Exchange, 1 serving:** 1 vegetable
**Calories, 1 serving:** 25

## Butternut Squash

| | | |
|---|---|---|
| 2 lbs. | butternut squash | 1 kg |
| 1 clove | garlic, minced | 1 clove |
| | water | |
| 2 T. | sesame seeds, toasted | 30 mL |
| 2 T. | wheat germ, toasted | 30 mL |
| | salt and pepper to taste | |

Wash and cut off stem of butternut squash; cut squash into thin slices and arrange in large skillet. Sprinkle with minced garlic. Add just enough water to steam the squash; cover and cook over medium heat. When squash is tender, drain off any excess water. Place on heated serving platter. Sprinkle with sesame seeds, wheat germ, salt and pepper.

**Yield:** 9 servings
**Exchange, 1 serving:** 2 vegetables
**Calories, 1 serving:** 42

## Best of Turnips

This is an easy and very flavorful recipe.

| | | |
|---|---|---|
| 2 slices | bacon | 2 slices |
| 2 lbs. | fresh turnips | 1 kg |

In a large skillet, fry bacon until crisp; remove from heat and crumble. Meanwhile, peel and finely grate the turnips. Place grated turnips in hot bacon fat. Toss and cook until turnips are well coated and slightly brown. Reduce heat; add a small amount of water to pan and cover tightly. Simmer on low heat until turnips are tender, about 25 to 30 minutes. Drain any remaining water or fat. Stir in crumbled bacon. Serve hot.

**Yield:** 6 servings
**Exchange, 1 serving:** 1 vegetable, ½ fat
**Calories, 1 serving:** 45

## Stewed Tomatoes & Green Beans

| | | |
|---|---|---|
| 2 cloves | garlic, minced | 2 cloves |
| 1 medium | onion, sliced into rings | 1 medium |
| ½ c. | green pepper, chopped | 125 mL |
| ½ c. | celery, sliced | 125 mL |
| 2 T. | low-cal margarine | 30 mL |
| 2 c. | fresh tomatoes, chopped | 500 mL |
| 2 c. | fresh green beans, snapped | 500 mL |
| | salt and pepper to taste | |

In a nonstick skillet, sauté garlic, onion rings, green pepper and celery in the margarine for 4 minutes. Add tomatoes, green beans, salt and pepper. Stir to mix. Reduce heat, cover and cook for about 15 minutes or until green beans are *al dente.*

**Yield:** 4 servings
**Exchange, 1 serving:** 2 vegetable
**Calories, 1 serving:** 50

# Soups & Stews

## Oriental Minestrone

| | | |
|---|---|---|
| 2 10¾-oz. cans | condensed chicken broth | 2 300-g cans |
| 1 | soup-can water | 1 |
| 2 oz. | uncooked spaghetti | 60 g |
| 1 clove | garlic, minced | 1 clove |
| 1 t. | ginger root, grated | 5 mL |
| 1 c. | carrots, cut into julienne slices | 250 mL |
| 1 c. | broccoli stems, thinly sliced, and small florets | 250 mL |
| | Wheat Germ Pork Balls (recipe follows) | |
| 1 c. | fresh pea pods, halved | 250 mL |
| 1 c. | fresh spinach, romaine lettuce or chard, chopped | 250 mL |

Heat together broth and water in a large saucepan until the boiling point. Stir in spaghetti, garlic and ginger. Bring to a boil. Cover and simmer for 6 minutes. Add carrots and broccoli. Cover and simmer for 2 to 3 minutes until vegetables are crisp-tender. Add Wheat Germ Pork Balls, pea pods and spinach, lettuce or chard. Heat thoroughly.

### WHEAT GERM PORK BALLS

| | | |
|---|---|---|
| ½ lb. | lean ground pork | 250 g |
| ¾ c. | Kretschmer regular wheat germ | 190 mL |
| ½ c. | water chestnuts, chopped | 125 mL |
| 2 T. | soy sauce | 30 mL |
| 2 T. | water | 30 mL |
| 1½ t. | ginger root, grated | 7 mL |
| dash | black pepper | dash |

Combine all ingredients. Shape into 24 balls. Place in a large, shallow baking pan. Bake at 400 °F (200 °C) for 20 minutes until lightly browned and thoroughly cooked. Cover and keep warm.

*Note*: ½ lb. (125 g) bulk pork sausage may be used instead of ground pork. Decrease soy sauce to 1 T. (15 mL) and increase water to 3 T. (45 mL).

**Microwave:** Prepare Wheat Germ Pork Balls as directed above. Place in 1½-qt. (1½-L) glass baking dish. Microwave on HIGH for 6 to 8 minutes or until meat is no longer pink, rotating once. Set aside. Place broth and water in a 3-qt. (3-L) glass casserole. Microwave on HIGH for 9 to 10 minutes or until liquid boils. Stir in spaghetti, garlic and ginger. Microwave on HIGH for 6 minutes. Add carrots and broccoli. Microwave on HIGH for 2 to 3 minutes or until vegetables are crisp-tender and spaghetti is tender. Add Wheat Germ Pork Balls, pea pods and spinach. Microwave on HIGH for 1½ to 2½ minutes or until pea pods are crisp-tender.

**Yield:** 6 servings
**Exchange, 1 serving:** 1 bread, 2 vegetable, 1 high-fat meat
**Calories, 1 serving:** 219

*With the courtesy of Kretschmer Wheat Germ/International Multifoods.*

# Gazpacho

| ¼ c. | *Mazola corn oil* | 60 mL |
|---|---|---|
| ½ c. | *onion, finely chopped* | 125 mL |
| 1 clove | *garlic, minced* | 1 clove |
| 1¼ c. | *tomato, peeled and chopped* | 310 mL |
| 1 c. | *green pepper, sliced into very thin strips* | 250 mL |
| ¼ c. | *fresh parsley, chopped* | 60 mL |
| dash | *hot pepper sauce* | dash |
| ¼ t. | *dried basil* | 1 mL |
| ¼ t. | *oregano* | 1 mL |
| dash | *black pepper* | dash |
| 1 | *cucumber, halved lengthwise, seeded and very thinly sliced* | 1 |
| ½ c. | *chicken broth* | 125 mL |
| ½ c. | *water* | 125 mL |
| ⅓ c. | *dry white wine* | 90 mL |

In a small saucepan, heat oil over medium heat. Add onion and garlic. Cook, stirring, for 2 minutes. In large bowl, stir together onion mixture and remaining ingredients.

**Yield:** 4 servings
**Exchange, 1 serving:** 2 vegetable, 1½ fat
**Calories, 1 serving:** 120

*"A Diet for the Young at Heart" by Mazola.*

## Cold Cucumber Soup

I happen to be a soup lover—so, a cold soup in summer is perfect.

| | | |
|---|---|---|
| 2 large | cucumbers | 2 large |
| 3 c. | water | 750 mL |
| 2 T. | cornstarch | 30 mL |
| 4 | chicken bouillon cubes | 4 |
| 1 T. | white wine vinegar | 15 mL |
| 1 T. | fresh dill, minced | 15 mL |
| ½ c. | Dannon low-fat plain yogurt | 125 mL |
| | salt and pepper to taste | |

Slice off ends of cucumbers; cut cucumbers into chunks. Combine 1 c. (250 mL) of the water and cucumber in blender or food processor. Mix together remaining water and cornstarch until blended. Combine cucumber and cornstarch mixtures in a large soup pot. Add bouillon cubes, vinegar and dill. Simmer and stir over low heat until bouillon cubes dissolve and mixture is hot. Remove from heat and cool slightly. Refrigerate, covered, until chilled. Stir in yogurt. Season with salt and pepper. Refrigerate until serving time.
**Yield:** 4 servings
**Exchange, 1 serving:** ⅓ nonfat milk
**Calories, 1 serving:** 31

## Spicy-Icy Tomato Soup

A cold soup with a snappy taste.

| | | |
|---|---|---|
| 2 lbs. | tomatoes | 1 kg |
| ½ c. | onion, diced | 125 mL |
| 1 t. | garlic, minced | 5 mL |
| 4-oz. can | green chilies, drained and chopped | 118-g can |
| 3 T. | whole wheat flour | 45 mL |
| 3 c. | chicken broth | 750 mL |
| ¼ t. | ground cumin | 1 mL |
| ¼ t. | ground coriander | 1 mL |
| ¼ t. | salt | 1 mL |
| ¼ t. | red pepper | 1 mL |
| | fresh parsley sprigs | |

Place tomatoes in blender or food processor and process until puréed. In a large saucepan or Dutch oven, heat oil and add onions, garlic and chilies. Cook and stir until onions are soft. Add flour and cook 1 minute longer, stirring constantly. Gradually stir in puréed tomatoes and chicken broth. Add cumin, coriander, salt and red pepper. Bring mixture to a boil. Reduce heat, cover and simmer for about 25 minutes, stirring occasionally, to prevent sticking. Remove from heat; cool to room temperature. Pour into large bowl or storage container. Refrigerate until thoroughly chilled. When serving the soup, garnish each bowl with a parsley sprig.

**Yield:** 7 c. (1¾ L)
**Exchange, 1 c. (250 mL):** 2 vegetable, 1 fat
**Calories, 1 c. (250):** 100

## Russian-Jewish Barley Soup

This recipe, given to me by my friend Sally Jordan, has been passed down through many generations of her family.

| | | |
|---|---|---|
| ¾ c. | *small lima beans* | 190 mL |
| 4 qts. | *water* | 4 L |
| 1½ lbs. | *neck or chuck soup bone* | 750 g |
| 1 c. | *celery, including leaves* | 250 mL |
| | *salt and pepper to taste* | |
| 1 | *onion, chopped* | 1 |
| 1 c. | *carrots, sliced* | 250 mL |
| 1 c. | *potatoes, diced* | 250 mL |
| ½ c. | *pearl barley* | 125 mL |

**Top of the stove method:** Place lima beans in mixing bowl, cover with 2 c. (500 mL) boiling water; soak overnight. In large soup pot, place soup bone, celery, onion and enough water to completely cover the bone. Season with salt and pepper. Bring to a boil, reduce heat and simmer until meat is very tender. Remove bone from soup pot arìd cut off all edible meat from the bone; return meat to the pot. Discard bone and membranes. Drain lima beans and add with the remaining ingredients to the soup pot. Adjust water to make 4 qts. (4 L) of soup. Taste and season with salt and pepper. Cover and simmer for 5 to 6 hours.

**Slow cooker method:** Place lima beans in mixing bowl, cover with 2 c. (500 mL) boiling water; soak overnight. In a slow cooker, place soup bone, celery, onion and enough water to completely cover bone. Add salt and pepper to taste. Cook on LOW during the night (8 to 12 hours). In the morning, remove meat from bone, discard bone and membranes. Drain lima beans and add with remaining ingredients to slow cooker. Add enough water to make 4 qts. (4 L) of soup. Adjust salt and pepper to taste.

**Yield:** 4 qts. (4 L)
**Exchange, 1 c. (250 mL):** 1 bread, ½ medium-fat meat
**Calories, 1 c. (250 mL):** 98

## Tortilla Soup

Tortilla soup is a Mexican classic. Most tortilla soups contain cheese, some include meat. Tortilla chips take the place of bread croutons in this recipe. Aficionados who like the hot flavor of Mexican foods can add ½ t. (2 mL) cayenne pepper to the blender ingredients.

| | | |
|---|---|---|
| 3 | tomatoes, peeled and cut in half | 3 |
| 1 medium | onion, coarsely chopped | 1 medium |
| 1 clove | garlic, minced | 1 clove |
| 2 T. | fresh parsley or coriander (cilantro), chopped | 30 mL |
| 15-oz. can | Health Valley tomato sauce | 450-g can |
| ¼ t. | honey | 1 mL |
| 2 13¾-oz. cans | Health Valley chicken broth | 2 390-g cans |
| 2 t. | Health Valley Instead of Salt all-purpose seasoning | 5 mL |
| 5½-oz. pkg. | Health Valley Buenitos tortilla chips | 150-g pkg. |
| 1 c. | cheddar cheese, grated | 250 mL |

In a blender, combine tomatoes, onion, garlic, parsley or coriander, tomato sauce and honey. Cover and blend until nearly smooth. Pour into a large saucepan. Stir in the broth and seasoning; bring to a boil, cover and simmer for 20 minutes. Divide tortilla chips among 5 soup bowls, sprinkle with cheese and pour hot soup into the bowls over the cheese. Serve immediately.

**Yield:** 5 servings
**Exchange, 1 serving:** 1 bread, 2 vegetable, 1 high-fat meat, 1 fat
**Calories, 1 serving:** 320

*From Health Valley Foods.*

## Meatball Vegetable Soup

| | | |
|---|---|---|
| 10½-oz. can | condensed beef broth soup | 300-g can |
| 4 c. | water | 1 L |
| 3½ c. | whole peeled tomatoes, not drained | 875 mL |
| 1¾ c. | cooked red kidney beans, not drained | 440 mL |
| 2 medium | onions, sliced | 2 medium |
| 1 c. | carrots, sliced | 250 mL |
| 1 clove | garlic, finely chopped | 1 clove |
| 1 t. | salt | 5 mL |
| ¼ t. | pepper | 1 mL |
| 1 t. | chili powder | 5 mL |

| ¾ c. | Kellogg's All-Bran cereal | 190 mL |
|---|---|---|
| 1 | egg, slightly beaten | 1 |
| dash | black pepper | dash |
| 1 lb. | lean ground beef | 500 g |
| 2 T. | vegetable oil | 30 mL |

In large saucepan or Dutch oven, combine 1 c. (250 mL) of the condensed soup, the water and next 8 ingredients, cutting tomatoes into pieces with a spoon. Bring to a boil. Reduce heat and simmer, uncovered, 30 minutes. Slightly crush the cereal. Mix with egg, remaining condensed soup and pepper. Add ground beef, mixing until thoroughly combined. Shape into 1-in. (2.5-cm) meatballs. Brown meatballs in heated oil. Drain. Add meatballs to vegetable mixture. Simmer, covered, about 30 minutes longer.

**Yield:** 12 servings
**Exchange, 1 serving:** 1 bread, 1 medium-fat meat
**Calories, 1 serving:** 150

*From Kellogg's Test Kitchens.*

## Krupnik

This is an American version of a very filling Polish soup. It is very tasty and quick to make.

| ½ c. | pearl barley | 125 mL |
|---|---|---|
| 2 qts. | water | 2 L |
| 6 | beef bouillon cubes | 6 |
| 16-oz. box | Green Giant frozen mixed vegetables | 457-g box |
| 2½-oz jar | Green Giant frozen sliced mushrooms | 72-g jar |
| 3 medium | potatoes, diced | 3 medium |
| 1 T. | fresh parsley, chopped | 15 mL |
| 2 t. | dillseed | 10 mL |
| 2 | egg yolks | 2 |

Cook barley as directed on package. Meanwhile, heat water and bouillon cubes in large soup kettle until cubes are dissolved. Add frozen vegetables, mushrooms, potatoes and 1 t. (5 mL) of the parsley and dillseed. Add the cooked barley. Beat egg yolks with a small amount of water. A little at a time, stir egg yolks into soup mixture. Pour into a large soup tureen. Garnish with the remaining parsley.

**Yield:** 6 servings
**Exchange, 1 serving:** 2 bread, ⅓ fat
**Calories, 1 serving:** 165

# Celebration Soup

| | | |
|---|---|---|
| 4 large | onions, thinly sliced | 4 large |
| 3 T. | butter | 45 mL |
| 6 c. | chicken broth | 1½ L |
| 14-oz. can | La Choy chop suey vegetables, rinsed and drained | 420-g can |
| | salt and pepper to taste | |

In saucepan, cook onions in butter for 5 minutes. Add 3 c. (750 mL) of the broth; simmer, covered, 15 minutes or until onions are tender. Stir in remaining broth and vegetables. Heat to serving temperature. Season with salt and pepper. Ladle into soup bowls.
**Yield:** 8 servings
**Exchange, 1 c.:** 1 vegetable, 1 fat
**Calories, 1 c.:** 62

*Adapted from a La Choy Food Products recipe.*

# Vegetable Chowder

| | | |
|---|---|---|
| 1 T. | Mazola corn oil | 15 mL |
| 1 medium | onion, sliced | 1 medium |
| ½ c. | celery, thinly sliced | 125 mL |
| 1 clove | garlic, minced | 1 clove |
| 2 c. | chicken broth | 500 mL |
| 16-oz. can | tomatoes, undrained and chopped | 470-g can |
| 1 c. | carrots, sliced | 250 mL |
| 1 t. | dried basil | 5 mL |
| ¼ t. | pepper | 1 mL |
| 20-oz. can | chick-peas, undrained | 500-g can |
| 12-oz. can | whole kernel corn, undrained | 360-g can |
| 1 c. | zucchini, sliced | 250 mL |

In 5-qt. (5-L) soup pot, heat oil over medium heat. Add onion, celery and garlic. Cook, stirring, 5 minutes or until tender. Add next 5 ingredients. Cook about 25 minutes or until carrots are crisp-tender. Add remaining ingredients and cook 15 to 20 minutes or until tender.
**Yield:** 8 servings
**Exchange, 1-c. (250-mL) serving:** 3 bread, ½ vegetable, ½ lean meat
**Calories, 1-c. (250-mL) serving:** 260

*"A Diet for the Young at Heart" by Mazola.*

# Fresh Pea Soup

A fast lunch.

| | | |
|---|---|---|
| 1 t. | vegetable oil | 5 mL |
| 1 c. | onion, chopped | 250 mL |
| 1 c. | carrots, shredded | 250 mL |
| 4 c. | iceberg lettuce, shredded | 1 L |
| 4 c. | fresh peas, shelled | 1 L |
| 8 c. | chicken broth | 2 L |
| 1 t. | salt | 5 mL |
| ½ t. | black pepper | 2 mL |

In a large soup pot or Dutch oven, heat oil over medium heat. Stir in the onion and carrots. Cover and cook 5 minutes or until onion is translucent but not brown. Add remaining ingredients and bring to a boil. Cover, reduce heat and simmer 10 to 15 minutes, stirring occasionally, until peas are tender. Remove from heat. Pour 2 c. (500 mL) of the soup into blender container. Cover and blend on low until mixture is puréed. Stir into the soup in the pot. Serve hot. (This soup freezes well for future use.)

**Yield:** 10 c. (2½ L)
**Exchange, 1 c. (250 mL):** ¾ bread
**Calories, 1 c. (250 mL):** 46

# Hamburger-Vegetable Chowder

| | | |
|---|---|---|
| ½ lb. | ground beef | 250 g |
| 1 c. | canned tomatoes | 250 mL |
| ½ c. | carrots, diced | 125 mL |
| ½ c. | celery, diced | 125 mL |
| 1 medium | onion, chopped | 1 medium |
| ½ t. | salt | 2 mL |
| ¼ t. | black pepper | 1 mL |
| ¼ c. | Stone-Buhr pearl barley | 60 mL |
| 1 c. | potatoes, cubed | 250 mL |
| 1½ qts. | water | 1½ L |

In a saucepan, slowly brown meat over low heat. Add remaining ingredients and simmer until barley is tender, about 1 hour; or cook in pressure cooker at 15 pounds pressure for about 15 minutes.

**Yield:** 4 servings
**Exchange, 1 serving:** 1 bread, 1 vegetable, 1½ medium-fat meat
**Calories, 1 serving:** 208

*With the compliments of Arnold Foods Company, Inc.*

## Green Bean Soup

When green beans are abundant in the summer, try this quick soup.

| | | |
|---|---|---|
| 3 c. | *green beans, cleaned and snapped* | *750 mL* |
| 3 c. | *chicken broth* | *750 mL* |
| 1 c. | *carrots, cleaned and grated* | *250 mL* |
| 3 | *green onions with tops, trimmed and chopped* | *3* |
| ½ t. | *salt* | *2 mL* |
| ⅓ c. | *Dannon low-fat plain yogurt* | *90 mL* |

Combine beans and 1 c. (250 mL) of broth in saucepan or Dutch oven. Bring to boil, reduce heat and simmer until beans are tender. Remove from heat. Pour 1 c. (250 mL) of beans mixture into blender. Purée, return to pan. Add carrots, green onions, remaining broth and salt to the soup. Simmer over low heat until mixture is hot. Remove from heat; stir in yogurt. Serve hot.

**Yield:** 6 servings
**Exchange, 1 serving:** 1 vegetable
**Calories, 1 serving:** 29

## Broccoli Soup

Broccoli is a good source of potassium and vitamins A and C. Always cook (steam, simmer or stir-fry) broccoli briefly—it should still have a firm texture and bright color when done.

| | | |
|---|---|---|
| 15-oz. can | *Health Valley potato soup* | *450-g can* |
| 13¾-oz. can | *Health Valley chicken broth* | *390-g can* |
| 10-oz. pkg. | *frozen broccoli spears, cut up* | *300-g pkg.* |
| dash | *ground or grated nutmeg* | *dash* |
| ½ t. | *garlic powder* | *2 mL* |
| ½ t. | *Health Valley Instead of Salt all-purpose seasoning* | *2 mL* |

Heat together potato soup and chicken broth. Cut broccoli into ¾-in. (19-mm) pieces, add to the soup and cook 5 minutes. Add seasonings. Serve piping hot.

**Yield:** 6 servings
**Exchange, 1 serving:** ¾ bread, 1 vegetable, ½ fat
**Calories, 1 serving:** 115

*From Health Valley Foods.*

## Lentil Soup

| | | |
|---|---|---|
| 2 T. | *Mazola corn oil* | *30 mL* |
| 1 c. | *onion, sliced* | *250 mL* |
| 1 clove | *garlic, minced* | *1 clove* |

| 4 c. | *water* | *1 L* |
|---|---|---|
| 14½-oz. can | *tomatoes* | *425-g can* |
| 1 c. | *lentils, rinsed, drained* | *250 mL* |
| 2 T. | *Worcestershire sauce* | *30 mL* |
| 1 c. | *carrots, thinly sliced* | *250 mL* |
| 1 T. | *lemon juice* | *15 mL* |
| 2 T. | *fresh parsley, chopped* | *30 mL* |
| | *peel of small lemon,* | |
| | *cut in very thin strips* | |

In 4-qt. (4-L) soup pot, heat oil over medium high heat. Add onion and garlic. Cook, stirring, 2 minutes or until tender. Add next 4 ingredients. Bring to a boil, reduce heat and simmer 1 to 1½ hours or until lentils are cooked. Add carrots and lemon juice during last 15 minutes. Garnish with parsley and lemon peel.

**Yield:** 6 c. (1½ L)
**Exchange, 1-c. (250-mL) serving:** 2 bread, 1 fat
**Calories, 1-c. (250-mL) serving:** 180

*"A Diet for the Young at Heart" by Mazola.*

## Beef Heart Stew

One of my family's favorites in the autumn.

| 1½ lbs. | *beef heart* | *750 g* |
|---|---|---|
| 2 t. | *salt* | *10 mL* |
| ¼ t. | *freshly ground black pepper* | *1 mL* |
| ½ c. | *celery, sliced* | *125 mL* |
| ½ c. | *carrots, sliced* | *125 mL* |
| 17-oz. can | *Green Giant golden whole kernel corn* | *484-g can* |
| 2 c. | *potatoes, sliced* | *500 mL* |
| 1 T. | *all-purpose flour* | *15 mL* |
| ½ c. | *cold water* | *125 mL* |

Clean beef heart by removing large tubes, fat and blood vessels. Place in a large saucepan or kettle, cover with water. Add salt, pepper and celery. Brint to a boil, reduce heat and simmer for 2 hours. Remove and slice the heart. Return sliced heart to pan; add carrots, corn and potatoes. Combine flour and water in bowl or shaker bottle; shake to blend thoroughly. Add to stew mixture. Cook and stir over medium heat until vegetables are crisp-tender and gravy thickens, adding additional water, if needed.

**Yield:** 8 servings
**Exchange, 1 serving:** 1 bread, 2 medium-fat meat
**Calories, 1 serving:** 218

## Lamb Kidney Stew

| | | |
|---|---|---|
| 6 | lamb kidneys | 6 |
| 1 qt. | water | 1 L |
| 1 t. | white vinegar | 5 mL |
| ½ c. | onions, chopped | 125 mL |
| 2 | green peppers, chopped | 2 |
| 1 c. | tomatoes, chopped | 250 mL |
| 2 T. | cornstarch | 30 mL |
| 1 c. | cooked kidney beans | 250 mL |
| 2 t. | salt | 10 mL |
| ½ t. | paprika | 2 mL |
| ½ t. | dried basil | 2 mL |
| ½ t. | dried thyme | 2 mL |

Clean kidneys and cut them into ½-in. (13-mm) pieces. Place in soup pot or Dutch oven. Add 3 c. (750 mL) of the water and vinegar. Bring to a boil, reduce heat and cover. Simmer for 1 hour or until tender. Add onion, green peppers and tomatoes and cook for 15 minutes. Dissolve cornstarch in remaining 1 c. (250 mL) water. Add to the stew and cook until mixture thickens. Add remaining ingredients and heat to the boiling point.

**Yield:** 8 servings
**Exchange, 1 serving:** ⅔ bread, 1 medium-fat meat
**Calories, 1 serving:** 125

## Blanco Gazpacho

| | | |
|---|---|---|
| 3 | tomatoes, cut in chunks | 3 |
| 1 large | cucumber, peeled and cut into 2-in. (5-cm) chunks | 1 large |
| 3 T. | onion, chopped | 45 mL |
| 1 slice | whole wheat bread | 1 slice |
| 2 c. | water | 500 mL |
| ½ c. | chicken broth | 125 mL |
| 2 T. | lemon juice | 30 mL |
| 1 clove | garlic | 1 clove |
| 1 t. | salt | 5 mL |
| ½ t. | black pepper | 2 mL |

Combine all ingredients in food processor fitted with the steel blade. Process on high speed, until mixture is smooth. Chill. Pour soup into bowls. Serve chilled. (This soup freezes well for future use.)

**Yield:** 4 c. (1 L)
**Exchange 1 c. (250 mL):** 1 vegetable
**Calories 1 c. (250 mL):** 40

## Italian Stew

| | | |
|---|---|---|
| 2 lbs. | stewing meat, cut in small pieces | 1 kg |
| ½ lb. | Hot Italian-Style Sausage (page 81) | 250 g |
| 2 c. | onions, diced | 500 mL |
| 1 T. | garlic, minced | 30 mL |
| ½ c. | dry red wine | 125 mL |
| 6 c. | eggplant, cut into 1-in. (2.5-cm) pieces | 1½ L |
| 4 c. | zucchini, cut into ½-in. (1.25-cm) pieces | 1 L |
| 2 c. | tomato sauce | 500 mL |
| 4 | tomatoes, cut in chunks | 4 |
| 2 t. | oregano | 10 mL |
| 1 t. | salt | 5 mL |
| ¼ t. | black pepper | 1 mL |
| ¼ t. | ground cinnamon | 1 mL |
| 1 c. | fresh parsley, chopped | 250 mL |

Place meats in a large soup pot or Dutch oven over medium heat. Cook and stir to brown the meat. When meat is browned, add onion and garlic and cook a few minutes longer, stirring until onion softens. Add wine; bring to a boil and simmer until most of the wine evaporates. Add eggplant, zucchini, tomato sauce, tomatoes, oregano, salt, pepper and cinnamon. Bring to a boil, reduce heat and simmer 30 to 40 minutes, stirring occasionally. Skim off and discard any fat. Stir in the parsley. Ladle into hot bowls. (This stew freezes well for future use.)
**Yield:** 11 c. (2¾ L)
**Exchange, 1 c. (250 mL):** 2 vegetable, 2 high-fat meat, 1 fat
**Calories, 1 c. (250 mL):** 295

## Crab Stew

| | | |
|---|---|---|
| 10-oz. can | tomato soup | 300-g can |
| 1½ c. | water | 375 mL |
| ½ c. | crab meat, flaked | 125 mL |
| ½ c. | bamboo shoots | 125 mL |
| ½ c. | mushrooms, sliced | 125 mL |
| ½ c. | brown rice, cooked | 125 mL |
| ⅓ c. | celery, sliced | 90 mL |
| ¼ c. | chive, chopped | 60 mL |
| | salt and pepper to taste | |

Combine all ingredients in a saucepan. Cook over low heat, stirring occasionally, until vegetables are tender. Serve hot.
**Yield:** 4 servings
**Exchange, 1 serving:** ½ bread, ½ vegetable, ½ lean meat
**Calories, 1 serving:** 79

## Savory Bean Stew

| | | |
|---|---|---|
| 1 c. | dry Stone-Buhr soybeans | 250 mL |
| 1 qt. | water | 1 L |
| ⅓ c. | onion, chopped | 90 mL |
| 1 T. | margarine | 15 mL |
| ½ lb. | ground beef | 250 g |
| 4 | tomatoes, cored but not peeled | 4 |
| | salt and pepper to taste | |

Wash beans and combine with the water in a soup pot. Boil for 2 minutes. Cover and let stand for 1 hour. Simmer 1 to 1½ hours or until almost tender, adding water if necessary. In a casserole or pan, brown onion in margarine. Add beef, stir and cook slowly for a few minutes. Cut tomatoes into small pieces. Combine all the ingredients. Simmer until meat is tender and the flavors are blended, about 45 to 50 minutes. Season with salt and pepper.

**Yield:** 5 servings
**Exchange, 1 serving:** 1 bread, 1½ medium-fat meat, 1 vegetable
**Calories, 1 serving:** 215

*With the compliments of Arnold Foods Company, Inc.*

## High Fiber Chili

| | | |
|---|---|---|
| 1 lb. | lean ground beef | 500 g |
| 1 large | onion, sliced | 1 large |
| ½ c. | green pepper, chopped | 125 mL |
| 2 c. | Kellogg's bran flakes cereal | 500 mL |
| 1 c. | tomato sauce | 250 mL |
| 1¾ c. | cooked red kidney beans, not drained | 440 mL |
| 2 c. | whole peeled tomatoes, not drained | 500 mL |
| ½ c. | water | 125 mL |
| 1 T. | chili powder | 15 mL |
| dash | garlic powder | dash |
| 1 t. | salt | 5 mL |
| 1 | bay leaf | 1 |

In a large saucepan, cook beef, onion and green pepper until meat is browned, stirring frequently. Drain off excess drippings. Stir in the remaining ingredients. Cover and simmer over low heat about 1 hour, stirring occasionally.

**Yield:** 6 servings
**Exchange, 1 serving:** 1 bread, 1 vegetable, 2 medium-fat meat
**Calories, 1 serving:** 242

*From Kellogg's Test Kitchens.*

# Sausages

## Sweet Pork & Raisin Bran Breakfast Sausage

| | | |
|---|---|---|
| ½ c. | ice-cold orange juice | 125 mL |
| ½ t. | celery flakes | 2 mL |
| ¼ t. | ground nutmeg | 1 mL |
| ¾ t. | ground black pepper | 4 mL |
| ½ t. | ground sage | 2 mL |
| ¾ t. | salt | 4 mL |
| ¼ t. | ground thyme | 1 mL |
| 1 lb. | freshly ground pork | 500 g |
| 1½ c. | raisin bran flakes | 375 mL |

Pour orange juice into a large bowl. Add seasonings and stir. Add ground pork and raisin bran flakes. Follow directions below.

**Yield:** 16 servings
**Exchange, 1 serving:** 1 medium-fat meat
**Calories, 1 serving:** 80

### DIRECTIONS FOR ALL SAUSAGES

Mix sausage the old-fashioned way with *clean hands* until *thoroughly* blended. Wrap sausage in plastic and refrigerate for several hours or overnight to allow herbs, spices and seasonings to permeate the meat. Sausage can be formed into patties or stuffed into natural casings, using standard stuffing procedures. Make 16 patties or links per recipe unless recipe specifies 8 patties or links. Fresh pork sausage should be refrigerated and used within a day or 2. Pan-fry or bake sausage until brown and juicy. *Pork must be cooked thoroughly.* Cooked or uncooked sausage can be individually wrapped with waxed paper, placed in a freezer bag and frozen for future use.

## Sweet Beef with Apples Breakfast Sausage

| | | |
|---|---|---|
| ½ c. | ice-cold apple juice | 125 mL |
| ½ t. | ground cinnamon | 2 mL |
| ½ t. | parsley flakes | 2 mL |
| ¼ t. | ground marjoram | 1 mL |
| ¾ t. | ground black pepper | 4 mL |
| ½ t. | ground sage | 2 mL |
| ¾ t. | salt | 4 mL |
| 1 lb. | freshly ground beef | 500 g |
| 1 c. | uncooked oatmeal | 250 mL |
| 3 T. | dried apple, diced | 45 mL |

Pour apple juice into large bowl. Add seasonings and stir. Add ground beef, oatmeal and dried apple. Mix sausage the old-fashioned way, following directions on page 73.
**Yield:** 16 servings
**Exchange, 1 serving:** 1 lean meat
**Calories, 1 serving:** 46

## Hot Pork Breakfast Sausage

| | | |
|---|---|---|
| 1 | egg | 1 |
| ¼ c. | ice-cold tomato juice | 60 mL |
| ¼ t. | ground allspice | 1 mL |
| ¼ t. | ground basil | 1 mL |
| ½ t. | parsley flakes | 2 mL |
| ¼ t. | ground ginger | 1 mL |
| 1 t. | ground paprika | 5 mL |
| ¾ t. | cayenne pepper | 4 mL |
| ¼ t. | cayenne pepper flakes | 1 mL |
| ½ t. | ground sage | 2 mL |
| ½ t. | salt | 4 mL |
| 1 lb. | freshly ground pork | 500 g |
| 1 c. | wheat germ | 250 mL |

In a large bowl, combine egg and tomato juice. Blend seasonings into the liquid. Add pork and wheat germ. Mix sausage the old-fashioned way, following directions on page 73.
**Yield:** 16 servings
**Exchange, 1 serving:** 1 high-fat meat
**Calories, 1 serving:** 93
*Added touch*: Although this is an excellent breakfast sausage, it's *great* at a picnic when grilled on an outdoor charcoal barbecue and served on a bun.

**Yield:** 8 servings
**Exchange, 1 serving:** 2 high-fat meat
**Calories, 1 serving:** 187
*Note*: Add exchanges and calories for bun and condiments.

## Hot Beef Breakfast Sausage

| | | |
|---|---|---|
| 1 | egg | 1 |
| ¼ c. | ice-cold mixed vegetable juice | 60 mL |
| ½ t. | celery seed | 2 mL |
| ¼ t. | ground mustard | 1 mL |
| ¼ t. | ground oregano | 1 mL |
| 1 t. | ground paprika | 5 mL |
| ½ t. | cayenne pepper | 2 mL |
| ½ t. | cayenne pepper flakes | 2 mL |
| ½ t. | ground sage | 2 mL |
| ½ t. | salt | 2 mL |
| 1 lb. | freshly ground beef | 500 g |
| 1½ c. | 40% bran flakes | 375 mL |

Combine egg and vegetable juice in a large bowl and blend in the seasonings. Add ground beef and bran flakes. Mix sausage the old-fashioned way, following directions on page 73.
**Yield:** 16 servings
**Exchange, 1 serving:** 1 lean-fat meat
**Calories, 1 serving:** 51
*Added touch*: Although this is an outstanding breakfast sausage, it is scrumptious at a picnic when grilled on an outdoor charcoal barbecue and served on a bun.
**Yield:** 8 servings
**Exchange, 1 serving:** 1 high-fat meat
**Calories, 1 serving:** 102
*Note*: Add exchanges and calories for bun and condiments.

## Sweet Minted Lamb Breakfast Sausage

| | | |
|---|---|---|
| ½ c. | ice-cold pineapple juice | 125 mL |
| ¼ t. | ground cinnamon | 1 mL |
| ½ t. | dried mint flakes | 2 mL |
| ¼ t. | ground marjoram | 1 mL |
| ¾ t. | ground black pepper | 4 mL |
| ¼ t. | ground rosemary | 1 mL |
| ½ t. | ground sage | 2 mL |
| ¾ t. | salt | 4 mL |

|         |                     |        |
|---------|---------------------|--------|
| ¼ t.    | ground thyme        | 1 mL   |
| 1 lb.   | freshly ground lamb  | 500 g  |
| 1 c.    | yellow cornmeal     | 250 mL |

In a large bowl, blend pineapple juice and seasonings. Add ground lamb and cornmeal. Mix the old-fashioned way, following directions on page 73.

**Yield:** 16 servings
**Exchange, 1 serving:** 1 lean meat
**Calories, 1 serving:** 53

## German-Style Bratwurst

Bratwurst is a plump traditional sausage that originated in Nürnberg, Germany. In the German language, *brat* means "to fry" and *wurst* means "sausage." Bratwurst, well-known throughout the world, is a common cookout favorite in the United States Midwest, especially in the Sheboygan/Milwaukee, Wisconsin area.

Bratwurst can be made of pork, beef and/or veal. There are countless ways to make bratwurst. Each sausage maker (*wurstmacher*) blends his or her own bratwurst variation, according to personal, regional and ethnic preferences. Bratwurst tastes best when charcoal-grilled and served with your favorite condiments on a German-style bun. The following bratwurst recipes are only a sampling of the hundreds of delightful variations that bratwurst fans have created. Although bratwurst is usually an all-meat sausage, these high-fiber variations retain the authentic style and flavor of the original recipes.

## Smoky-Style Pork Bratwurst

|         |                          |        |
|---------|--------------------------|--------|
| 1       | egg                      | 1      |
| ¼ c.    | ice water                | 60 mL  |
| 1 t.    | liquid smoke             | 5 mL   |
| 1 t.    | caraway seeds            | 5 mL   |
| ½ t.    | celery flakes            | 2 mL   |
| ¼ t.    | parsley flakes           | 1 mL   |
| ¼ t.    | ground ginger            | 1 mL   |
| ½ t.    | ground dry orange peel   | 2 mL   |
| ¼ t.    | ground nutmeg            | 1 mL   |
| 1 t.    | onion powder             | 5 mL   |
| ½ t.    | ground white pepper      | 2 mL   |
| ¾ t.    | salt                     | 4 mL   |
| ¼ t.    | brown sugar              | 1 mL   |

| 1 lb. | freshly ground pork | 500 g |
| 1¼ c. | 40% bran flakes | 310 mL |

In a large bowl, combine the egg, water and liquid smoke. Crush caraway seeds, celery and parsley flakes with a mortar and pestle. Blend all seasonings into the liquid. Add pork and bran flakes. Mix sausage the old-fashioned way, following directions on page 73. Make eight patties or links per recipe.

*Added touch*: Bake fresh or frozen bratwurst with sauerkraut for a delectable main dish.

**Yield:** 8 servings

**Exchange, 1 serving:** 2 medium-fat meat

**Calories, 1 serving:** 151

## Smoky-Style Beef & Pork Bratwurst

| 1 | egg | 1 |
| 1 t. | liquid smoke | 5 mL |
| ¼ c. | ice water | 60 mL |
| ¼ t. | allspice | 1 mL |
| ½ t. | caraway seeds | 2 mL |
| 1½ t. | celery flakes | 7 mL |
| ¼ t. | ground ginger | 1 mL |
| 1 t. | ground dry lemon peel | 5 mL |
| ¼ t. | ground mace | 1 mL |
| 1 t. | onion flakes | 5 mL |
| ¾ t. | ground black pepper | 4 mL |
| ¾ t. | salt | 4 mL |
| dash | brown sugar | dash |
| ½ lb. | freshly ground beef | 250 g |
| ½ lb. | freshly ground pork | 250 g |
| 1 c. | wheat germ | 250 mL |

Add egg, liquid smoke and water to large bowl. Crush caraway seeds and celery flakes in a mortar with pestle. Blend seasonings into the liquid. Add beef, pork and wheat germ. Mix sausage the old-fashioned way, following directions on page 73. Make 8 patties or links per recipe.

*Added touch*: Use diced, sliced or crumbled bratwurst as a pizza topping.

**Yield:** 8 servings

**Exchange, 1 serving:** 2 medium-fat meat

**Calories, 1 serving:** 169

*Note:* Add exchanges and calories of pizza dough and other toppings.

## Spicy Beef Bratwurst

| 1 | egg | 1 |
|---|---|---|
| ¼ c. | cold milk | 60 mL |
| ¼ t. | caraway seeds | 1 mL |
| 1 t. | parsley flakes | 5 mL |
| ¼ t. | ground coriander | 1 mL |
| 1 t. | ground dry lemon peel | 5 mL |
| ¼ t. | ground mace | 1 mL |
| ¼ t. | ground mustard | 1 mL |
| 1 T. | onion or leek, diced | 15 mL |
| 1 T. | onion powder | 15 mL |
| ¼ t. | paprika | 1 mL |
| ¾ t. | ground white pepper | 4 mL |
| 1 t. | salt | 5 mL |
| ¼ t. | brown sugar | 1 mL |
| 1 lb. | freshly ground beef | 500 g |
| 1 c. | uncooked oatmeal | 250 mL |

Combine egg and milk in a large bowl. Crush caraway seeds and parsley flakes in mortar with pestle. Blend all seasonings into the liquid. Add beef and oatmeal. Mix sausage the old-fashioned way, following directions on page 73. Make 8 patties or links per recipe.
**Yield:** 8 servings
**Exchange, 1 serving:** 1 high-fat meat
**Calories, 1 serving:** 119

## Veal & Pork Bratwurst

| 1 | egg | 1 |
|---|---|---|
| ¼ c. | ice water | 60 mL |
| ¾ t. | caraway seeds | 4 mL |
| ½ t. | celery seeds | 2 mL |
| ¼ t. | allspice | 1 mL |
| ¼ t. | ground coriander | 1 mL |
| ¾ t. | ground dry lemon peel | 4 mL |
| ¼ t. | ground nutmeg | 1 mL |
| ¾ t. | onion powder or flakes | 4 mL |
| ½ t. | parsley flakes | 2 mL |
| ¾ t. | ground black pepper | 4 mL |
| 1 t. | salt | 5 mL |
| ½ lb. | freshly ground veal | 250 g |
| ½ lb. | freshly ground pork | 250 g |
| 1 c. | Kellogg's All-Bran cereal | 250 mL |

In a large bowl, mix the egg and water. Crush caraway and celery seeds in a mortar with pestle. Blend seasonings into the liquid. Add veal, pork and cereal. Mix sausage the old-fashioned way, following directions on page 73. Make 8 patties or links per recipe. Bratwurst should be refrigerated and used within a day or 2.

**Yield:** 8 servings
**Exchange, 1 serving:** 2 medium-fat meat
**Calories, 1 serving:** 139

## Viennese-Style Sausage

Viennese-Style Sausage is delightful when smothered in hot tomato sauce and served as an appetizer or as the meat in your favorite casserole.

| | | |
|---|---|---|
| ½ c. | *ice-cold milk* | *125 mL* |
| 1 T. | *all-purpose flour* | *15 mL* |
| ½ t. | *ground coriander* | *2 mL* |
| ¼ t. | *ground mace* | *1 mL* |
| 1 T | *onion, diced* | *15 mL* |
| ½ t. | *ground paprika* | *2 mL* |
| ¼ t. | *cayenne pepper* | *1 mL* |
| 1 t. | *salt* | *5 mL* |
| ¼ t. | *sugar* | *1 mL* |
| ½ lb. | *freshly ground beef* | *250 g* |
| ½ lb. | *freshly ground pork* | *250 g* |
| 1 c. | *white cornmeal* | *250 mL* |

Pour milk into a quart (liter) jar. Sprinkle flour into the jar, cover and shake to blend. Pour milk and flour solution into a large bowl. Blend seasonings into the liquid. Add beef, pork and cornmeal. Mix sausage the old-fashioned way, following directions on page 73.

**Yield:** 16 servings
**Exchange, 1 serving:** 1⅔ high-fat meat
**Calories, 1 serving:** 173
*Note*: Add exchanges and calories for all other foods used with Viennese-Style Sausage.

## Parisienne-Style Sausage

| | | |
|---|---|---|
| ½ c. | *Burgundy wine, chilled* | *125 mL* |
| 1 T. | *white flour* | *15 mL* |
| ¼ t. | *ground bay leaf* | *1 mL* |
| ¼ t. | *ground clove* | *1 mL* |
| ¼ t. | *ground coriander* | *1 mL* |
| ¼ t. | *ground ginger* | *1 mL* |
| ¼ t. | *ground mace* | *1 mL* |
| ½ t. | *ground nutmeg* | *2 mL* |
| 1 t. | *ground black pepper* | *5 mL* |

| 1¼ t. | salt | 6 mL |
|---|---|---|
| ½ t. | ground savory | 2 mL |
| ¼ t. | sugar | 1 mL |
| ¼ t. | ground tarragon | 1 mL |
| ¼ t. | ground thyme | 1 mL |
| ½ lb. | freshly ground pork | 250 g |
| ½ lb. | freshly ground beef | 250 g |
| 1 c. | yellow cornmeal | 250 mL |

Pour chilled wine into a large bowl. Blend flour and seasonings into the wine. Add pork, beef and cornmeal. Mix sausage the old-fashioned way, following directions on page 73.
**Yield:** 16 servings
**Exchange, 1 serving:** 1 medium-fat meat
**Calories, 1 serving:** 66

## Greek-Style Loukanika

Loukanika can be served as a main dish for dinner or on Greek-style bread as a luncheon meal.

| ½ c. | rosé wine, chilled | 125 mL |
|---|---|---|
| 2 T. | orange juice, chilled | 30 mL |
| ¼ t. | ground allspice | 1 mL |
| ¼ t. | ground cinnamon | 1 mL |
| ¼ t. | ground cumin | 1 mL |
| 1 clove | garlic, minced | 1 clove |
| ¼ t. | ground nutmeg | 1 mL |
| 2 T. | orange peel, grated | 30 mL |
| ¼ t. | ground black pepper | 1 mL |
| ½ t. | peppercorns, cracked | 2 mL |
| 1 t. | salt | 5 mL |
| 1 t. | dried savory | 5 mL |
| ¼ t. | brown sugar | 1 mL |
| ½ lb. | freshly ground veal | 250 g |
| ½ lb. | freshly ground pork | 250 g |
| 1 c. | bulgur | 250 mL |

Mix wine and orange juice in a large bowl. Blend all seasonings into the liquid. Add veal, pork and bulgur. Mix sausage the old-fashioned way, following directions on page 73. Make 8 patties or links per recipe.
**Yield:** 8 servings
**Exchange, 1 serving:** 2 medium-fat meat
**Calories, 1 serving:** 139
*Note:* Add exchanges and calories for all other foods used with loukanika.

# Italian-Style Sausage

Italian sausage is a worldwide favorite. Sweet or hot Italian sausage can be served as a main dish, on a slice of hot Italian bread, as the meat sauce on spaghetti or as a pizza topping. Use your imagination to create delightful menus using the following delicious sausages.

## Sweet Italian-Style Sausage

| | | |
|---|---|---|
| ½ c. | ice water | 125 mL |
| ¾ t. | aniseed | 4 mL |
| ½ t. | ground coriander | 2 mL |
| ½ t. | ground paprika | 2 mL |
| ¼ t. | ground black pepper | 1 mL |
| ¼ t. | ground cayenne pepper | 1 mL |
| ¼ t. | cayenne pepper flakes | 1 mL |
| ¾ t. | salt | 4 mL |
| ¼ t. | brown sugar | 1 mL |
| 1 lb. | freshly ground pork | 500 g |
| 1 c. | bulgur | 250 mL |

Pour ice water into a large bowl. Crush aniseed with mortar and pestle. Blend seasonings into the liquid. Add pork and bulgur. Mix sausage the old-fashioned way, following directions on page 73. Make 8 patties or links per recipe.

**Yield:** 8 servings
**Exchange, 1 serving:** 1½ high-fat meat
**Calories, 1 serving:** 156

## Hot Italian-Style Sausage

| | | |
|---|---|---|
| ½ c. | dry Italian red wine | 125 mL |
| ½ t. | fennel seed | 2 mL |
| 1 t. | liquid smoke | 5 mL |
| 1 t. | paprika | 5 mL |
| 1 t. | cayenne pepper | 5 mL |
| ¾ t. | cayenne pepper flakes | 4 mL |
| 1 t. | salt | 5 mL |
| 1 lb. | freshly ground pork | 500 g |
| 1 c. | 40% bran flakes | 250 mL |

Chill the wine. Pour into a large bowl. Crush fennel seed with mortar and pestle. Blend all seasonings into the liquid. Add pork and 40% bran flakes. Mix sausage the old-fashioned way, following directions on page 73. Make 8 patties or links per recipe.

**Yield:** 8 servings
**Exchange, 1 serving:** 2 medium-fat meat
**Calories, 1 serving:** 151

## Luganega—Northern Italian-Style Sausage

| | | |
|---|---|---|
| ½ c. | Italian white vermouth | 125 mL |
| 2 T. | orange juice | 30 mL |
| 4 T. | Parmesan cheese, grated | 45 mL |
| ¼ t. | ground coriander | 1 mL |
| 1 clove | garlic, minced | 1 clove |
| ¼ t. | ground dry lemon peel | 1 mL |
| ¼ t. | ground nutmeg | 1 mL |
| ¼ t. | ground dry orange peel | 1 mL |
| ¼ t. | ground black pepper | 1 mL |
| ¾ t. | salt | 4 mL |
| 1 lb. | freshly ground pork | 500 g |
| 1 c. | wheat germ | 250 mL |

Chill vermouth and pour into a large bowl. Blend seasonings into the liquid. Add pork and wheat germ. Mix sausage the old-fashioned way, following directions on page 73. Make 8 patties or links per recipe.

**Yield:** 8 servings
**Exchange, 1 serving:** 2 high-fat meat
**Calories, 1 serving:** 188

## Near Eastern-Style Sausage

Serve as a main meat dish, baked with your favorite casserole or on pita bread with condiments.

| | | |
|---|---|---|
| ½ c. | ice water | 125 mL |
| dash | ground allspice | dash |
| ¼ t. | ground cloves | 1 mL |
| 2 cloves | garlic, minced | 2 cloves |
| ¼ t. | ground oregano | 1 mL |
| ½ t. | ground black pepper | 2 mL |
| ½ t. | ground rosemary | 2 mL |
| 1 t. | salt | 5 mL |
| ¼ t. | sugar | 1 mL |
| 1 lb. | freshly ground lamb | 500 g |
| 1 c. | bran flakes | 250 mL |

Pour ice water into a large bowl. Blend seasonings into the liquid. Add lamb and bran flakes. Mix sausage the old-fashioned way, following directions on page 73. Make 8 patties or links per recipe.

**Yield:** 8 servings
**Exchange, 1 serving:** 1 high-fat meat or 2 lean meat
**Calories, 1 serving:** 118

*Note*: Add calories and exchanges for condiments or other foods served with Near Eastern-Style Sausage.

# Polish-Style Sausage

Polish-style sausage, a favorite throughout the Western World, can be served on a whole wheat or rye bun with your favorite condiments. This sausage is great as a main dish all by itself or cooked with sauerkraut. You can be creative and develop your own favorite menus featuring Polish-style sausage.

## Mild Polish-Style Sausage

| | | |
|---|---|---|
| ½ c. | ice water | 125 mL |
| ¼ t. | celery seed | 1 mL |
| ½ t. | garlic powder | 2 mL |
| ½ t. | ground marjoram | 1 mL |
| dash | ground or grated nutmeg | dash |
| ½ t. | ground black pepper | 2 mL |
| 1 t. | salt | 5 mL |
| ¼ t. | brown sugar | 1 mL |
| ¼ t. | ground thyme | 1 mL |
| ½ lb. | freshly ground beef | 250 g |
| ½ lb. | freshly ground pork | 250 g |
| 1 c. | 40% bran flakes | 250 mL |

Pour water into a large bowl. Blend seasonings into the liquid. Add beef, pork and bran flakes. Mix sausage the old-fashioned way, following directions on page 73. Make 8 patties or links per recipe.

**Yield:** 8 servings
**Exchange, 1 serving:** 2 medium-fat meat
**Calories, 1 serving:** 122

## Spicy Polish-Style Sausage

| | | |
|---|---|---|
| ½ c. | ice-cold beer | 125 mL |
| 1 t. | liquid smoke | 5 mL |
| ¼ t. | ground allspice | 1 mL |
| ½ t. | celery seed | 2 mL |
| ¼ t. | ground coriander | 1 mL |
| 2 cloves | garlic, minced | 2 cloves |
| ½ t. | ground marjoram | 2 mL |
| ¼ t. | ground mace | 1 mL |
| 1 t. | ground paprika | 5 mL |
| 1 t. | ground white pepper | 5 mL |
| ¾ t. | salt | 4 mL |
| ½ t. | ground thyme | 2 mL |
| ¼ lb. | freshly ground beef | 125 g |
| ¾ lb. | freshly ground pork | 375 g |
| 1 c. | bulgur | 250 mL |

Pour beer into a large bowl. Blend seasonings into the beer. Add beef, pork, and bulgur. Mix sausage the old-fashioned way, following directions on page 73. Make 8 patties or links per recipe.
**Yield:** 8 servings
**Exchange, 1 serving:** 1½ high-fat meat
**Calories, 1 serving:** 147

## Russian-Style Kielbasa

| | | |
|---|---|---|
| ½ c. | ice water | 125 mL |
| 1 t. | vinegar | 5 mL |
| ¼ t. | dillseed | 1 mL |
| ¼ t. | ground allspice | 1 mL |
| ¼ t. | celery flakes | 1 mL |
| ¼ t. | cinnamon | 1 mL |
| 2 cloves | garlic, minced | 2 cloves |
| ½ t. | ground marjoram | 2 mL |
| ¼ t. | paprika | 1 mL |
| 1 t. | ground black pepper | 5 mL |
| ¾ t. | salt | 4 mL |
| 1 lb. | freshly ground beef | 500 g |
| ½ c. | oatmeal | 125 mL |
| ½ c. | wheat germ | 125 mL |

Combine water and vinegar in a large bowl. Crack dillseed in a mortar and pestle. Blend seasonings into the liquid. Add beef, oatmeal and wheat germ. Mix sausage the old-fashioned way, following directions on page 73. Make 8 patties or links per recipe.
**Yield:** 8 servings
**Exchange, 1 serving:** 1¼ high-fat meat
**Calories, 1 serving:** 126
*Note:* Add calories and exchanges for condiments or other foods served with Russian-Style Kielbasa.

## Scandinavian-Style Potato Sausage

Scandinavian-Style Potato Sausage can be served on a bun with condiments, as a meat entrée or as the meat in a delicious stew.

| | | |
|---|---|---|
| ¼ c. | ice-cold milk | 60 mL |
| 1 | egg | 1 |
| ¼ t. | allspice | 1 mL |
| dash | ground mace | dash |
| ¼ t. | ground nutmeg | 1 mL |
| 4 T. | onion, minced | 60 mL |
| 1 t. | ground black pepper | 5 mL |
| 1 t. | salt | 5 mL |
| ¼ t. | brown sugar | 1 mL |

| ½ lb. | freshly ground beef | 250 g |
| ½ lb. | freshly ground pork | 250 g |
| ½ c. | bran flakes | 125 mL |
| ½ c. | dried instant potatoes | 125 mL |

Combine egg and milk in a large bowl. Blend seasonings into the liquid. Add beef, pork, bran flakes and potatoes. Mix sausage the old-fashioned way, following directions on page 73. Make 8 patties or links per recipe.

**Yield:** 8 servings
**Exchange, 1 serving:** 1½ high-fat meat or 2 medium-fat meat
**Calories, 1 serving:** 143

## Spanish-Style Chorizo

Chorizo is prized throughout the Spanish-speaking world. Serve spicy or hot chorizo as a main dish on a slice of hot bread or as the meat in a Spanish or Mexican dish. Use your imagination to create delightful menus using chorizo.

### Spicy Spanish-Style Chorizo

| ½ c. | ice water | 125 mL |
| 1 T. | cider vinegar | 15 mL |
| ½ t. | aniseed | 2 mL |
| ¼ t. | chili powder | 1 mL |
| ¼ t. | ground cumin | 1 L |
| ½ t. | garlic powder | 2 mL |
| 1 t. | ground marjoram | 5 mL |
| 2 T. | onion, minced | 30 mL |
| ½ t. | ground paprika | 2 mL |
| ¼ t. | ground black pepper | 1 mL |
| ½ t. | cayenne pepper | 2 mL |
| ½ t. | cayenne pepper flakes | 2 mL |
| 1 t. | salt | 5 mL |
| ¼ t. | brown sugar | 1 mL |
| 1 lb. | freshly ground pork | 500 g |
| 1 c. | yellow cornmeal | 250 mL |

Combine water and vinegar in a large bowl. Crush aniseed with mortar and pestle. Blend seasonings into the liquid. Add pork and cornmeal. Mix sausage the old-fashioned way, following directions on page 73. Make 8 patties or links per recipe.

**Yield:** 8 servings
**Exchange, 1 serving:** 2 high-fat meat
**Calories, 1 serving:** 180

## Hot Spanish-Style Chorizo

| | | |
|---|---|---|
| ½ c. | red wine, chilled | 125 mL |
| 1 T. | cider vinegar | 15 mL |
| 1 t. | dark corn syrup | 5 mL |
| ½ t. | fennel seed | 2 mL |
| 1 t. | chili powder | 5 mL |
| ½ t. | ground cumin | 2 mL |
| 2 cloves | garlic, minced | 2 cloves |
| 1 T. | onion powder | 15 mL |
| 1 t. | ground oregano | 5 mL |
| 2 t. | ground paprika | 10 mL |
| 1 t. | cayenne pepper | 5 mL |
| 1 t. | cayenne pepper flakes | 5 mL |
| ¾ t. | salt | 4 mL |
| 1 lb. | freshly ground pork | 500 g |
| 1 c. | wheat germ | 250 mL |

Mix wine, vinegar and corn syrup in a large mixing bowl. Crush fennel seed in mortar with pestle. Blend seasonings into the liquid. Add pork and wheat germ. Mix sausage the old-fashioned way, following directions on page 73. Make 8 patties or links per recipe.

**Yield:** 8 servings
**Exchange, 1 serving:** 2 high-fat meat
**Calories, 1 serving:** 196

# Entrées

## Louis's Seafood Surprise

I really had trouble placing this recipe in the cookbook. I suppose it should go in soups and stews. But it is so good—I figured, "what the hay, let's put it with the Entrées."

| | | |
|---|---|---|
| 3 | tomatoes | 3 |
| ⅓ c. | fresh green beans | 90 mL |
| ½ can | tomato soup | ½ can |
| 3 c. | water | 750 mL |
| 1 c. | celery, chopped | 250 mL |
| 1 c. | carrots, grated | 250 mL |
| 1 c. | mushrooms, sliced | 250 mL |
| ½ c. | cabbage, shredded | 125 mL |
| ½ c. | onion, chopped | 125 mL |
| ¼ c. | corn | 60 mL |
| ¼ c. | peas | 60 mL |
| 1 clove | garlic, finely chopped | 1 clove |
| 2 t. | salt | 10 mL |
| ½ t. | dried basil | 2 mL |
| ½ t. | parsley flakes | 2 mL |
| ¼ t. | dried marjoram | 1 mL |
| ¼ t. | ground red pepper | 1 mL |
| ½ lb. | sole, cut into bite-size pieces | 250 g |
| 4 oz. | small shrimp | 120 g |
| 4 oz. | crab meat, cut into bite-size pieces | 120 g |

Core but do not peel tomatoes; cut into medium-size pieces. Clean and snap beans. Combine tomato soup, water and all vegetables in large saucepan. Add salt, basil, parsley flakes, sweet marjoram and red pepper. Cover tightly and cook over low heat until tomatoes are soft. Add sole, shrimp and crab. Cook until sole is firm but not broken. Serve in heated soup bowls.

**Yield:** 8 servings
**Exchange, 1 serving:** ½ bread, 1 medium-fat meat
**Calories, 1 serving:** 99

## Crab a la Lourna

This easy but elegant dinner was served the night our friend Lourna
came to dinner.

| | | |
|---|---|---|
| 2 T. | unsalted butter | 30 mL |
| ½ lb. | small snow-white mushrooms | 250 g |
| ½ lb. | snow peas | 250 g |
| ½ lb. | crab meat, cut into bite-size pieces | 250 g |
| 1 T. | all-purpose flour | 15 mL |
| 1 t. | cornstarch | 5 mL |
| 1 c. | cold water | 250 mL |
| ½ c. | 2% milk | 125 mL |
| | salt and pepper to taste | |
| 1 c. | wild rice, cooked | 250 mL |
| 2 c. | brown rice, cooked | 500 mL |

Heat a large skillet and melt 1 T. (15 mL) of the butter. Add mushrooms
and sauté until tender; remove from heat. Meanwhile, clean snow peas
and cut into 1-in. (2.5-cm) pieces. With a slotted spoon, remove mushrooms from skillet and return pan to medium heat. Add snow peas and
cook until peas are tender; remove peas from pan. Melt remaining 1 T.
(15 mL) butter. Add crab meat and sauté until lightly browned. Remove
from pan. Dissolve flour and cornstarch in the water. Pour into skillet,
add milk and simmer over low heat until mixture thickens. Season
with salt and pepper. Return mushrooms, peas and crab, heat and fold
mixture gently until hot. Combine hot wild and brown rice. Serve Crab
a la Lourna over the hot rice.

**Yield:** 6 servings
**Exchange, 1 serving:** 1 bread, 1 vegetable, 1 medium-fat meat
**Calories, 1 serving:** 178

## Crab Fried Rice

| | | |
|---|---|---|
| 2 T. | margarine | 30 mL |
| 2 | eggs, lightly beaten | 2 |
| 1 c. | mushrooms, sliced | 250 mL |
| 1 c. | celery, sliced | 250 mL |
| ½ c. | onion, chopped | 125 mL |
| ¼ c. | bamboo shoots | 60 mL |
| ¼ c. | water chestnuts, sliced | 60 mL |
| 3 c. | brown rice, cooked | 750 mL |
| 3 T. | soy sauce | 45 mL |
| ½ lb. | crab meat, cut in chunks | 500 g |
| | salt and pepper, if needed | |

Melt 1 T. (15 mL) of the margarine in a large nonstick skillet. Add eggs
and cook over low heat until set; remove to cutting board. Chop or cut

eggs into large strips. Melt remaining 1 T. (15 mL) margarine in the same pan. Add vegetables, cook and stir until celery is tender. Remove vegetables from pan. Stir the rice into pan and add soy sauce. Mix until completely blended. Add vegetables, crab and egg. Cover and cook over low heat until mixture is hot.

**Yield:** 6 servings
**Exchange, 1 serving:** 1 bread, 1 vegetable, 1 medium-fat meat
**Calories, 1 serving:** 176

## Tuna Patties

| | | |
|---|---|---|
| 2 | eggs | 2 |
| 2 6½-oz. cans | chunk light tuna in water | 2 185-g cans |
| ⅓ c. | milk | 90 mL |
| dash | pepper | dash |
| 1 t. | lemon juice | 5 mL |
| 2 T. | pickle relish | 30 mL |
| 1 c. | Kellogg's bran flakes cereal | 250 mL |
| | fresh parsley, snipped | |

Beat eggs lightly. Add remaining ingredients except parsley. Mix well. Shape into 6 patties. Place on lightly greased baking sheet. Bake at 350 °F (175 °C) about 25 minutes, turning patties after 15 minutes. Sprinkle with parsley.

**Yield:** 6 servings
**Exchange, 1 serving:** 2 lean meat, ⅓ bread
**Calories, 1 serving:** 125

*Based on a recipe from Kellogg's Test Kitchens.*

## Soy Flour Meat Loaf

| | | |
|---|---|---|
| 1 lb. | ground meat | 500 g |
| 2 | eggs | 2 |
| 1 c. | milk | 250 mL |
| 2½ t. | salt | 12 mL |
| ½ c. | Stone-Buhr soy flour | 125 mL |
| ¼ c. | Stone-Buhr quick-cooking rolled oats | 60 mL |
| ½ c. | onion, minced | 125 mL |
| ¼ t. | black pepper | 1 mL |

Combine all ingredients and mix well. Shape the loaf and place in a 9 × 5-in. (23 × 13-cm) loaf pan. Bake at 350 °F (175 °C) for 50 minutes or until done.

**Yield:** 6 servings
**Exchange, 1 serving:** ¾ bread, 2 medium-fat meat
**Calories, 1 serving:** 217

*With the compliments of Arnold Foods Company, Inc.*

## Slim Eggplant Parmigiana

| | | |
|---|---|---|
| 8 slices | eggplant, ¼-in. (6-mm) thick | 8 slices |
| 1 T. | Mazola corn oil | 15 mL |
| 8 t. | Corn Oil Herb Blend (recipe follows) | 40 mL |
| 4 oz. | skim-milk mozzarella cheese, thinly sliced | 120 g |
| 8 slices | tomato | 8 slices |
| 4 t. | Parmesan cheese, grated | 20 mL |

Lightly brush 1 side of eggplant slices with oil. On a cookie sheet, place eggplant slices with the oil side down. Spread top of each eggplant slice with 1 T. (15 mL) of the herb mixture. Top with mozzarella, tomato and cheese. Bake at 375 °F (190 °C) for 15 minutes or until eggplant is tender.

### CORN OIL HERB BLEND

| | | |
|---|---|---|
| ¼ c. | Mazola corn oil | 60 mL |
| 1 c. | fresh parsley | 250 mL |
| 1 t. | dried basil | 5 mL |
| 1 t. | dried marjoram | 5 mL |
| dash | black pepper | dash |

In blender container, place the corn oil, parlsey, basil, marjoram and pepper; cover. Blend on medium speed 1 minute or until smooth.
**Yield:** 4 servings
**Exchange, 1 serving:** 1 vegetable, 1½ high-fat meat
**Calories, 1 serving:** 210

*"A Diet for the Young at Heart" by Mazola.*

## Stuffed Eggplant Italiano

| | | |
|---|---|---|
| 1 lb. | eggplant | 500 g |
| ⅓ c. | All-Bran cereal | 90 mL |
| 1 c. | fresh mushrooms, sliced | 250 mL |
| ¼ c. | Parmesan cheese, grated | 60 mL |
| ¼ c. | onion, chopped | 60 mL |
| ¼ c. | green pepper, finely chopped | 60 mL |
| 2 T. | margarine, melted | 30 mL |
| 1 small clove | garlic, finely chopped | 1 small clove |
| ½ t. | salt | 2 mL |
| ½ t. | dried basil | 2 mL |
| dash | black pepper | dash |
| ⅓ c. | mozzarella cheese, shredded | 90 mL |

Cut eggplant in half lengthwise. Place halves, cut side down, in shallow baking pan. Bake at 350 °F (175 °C) for 15 minutes. Remove from oven. Cool slightly. Scoop out pulp, leaving ⅜-in. (1-cm) shell. Place shells, cut side up, in baking pan. Coarsely chop eggplant pulp. Combine with remaining ingredients except mozzarella cheese. Fill eggplant shells, pressing firmly. Cover with foil. Pierce foil in several places to allow steam to escape. Bake at 350 °F (175 °C) about 40 minutes or until vegetables are tender. Remove foil and sprinkle with the mozzarella. Bake, uncovered, about 2 minutes longer or until cheese melts. Cut each half into 2 pieces to serve.

**Yield:** 4 servings
**Exchange, 1 serving:** 2 medium-fat meat
**Calories, 1 serving:** 150

*From Kellogg's Test Kitchens.*

## Curried Veal with Rice

| | | |
|---|---|---|
| 4 T. | *Mazola corn oil* | *60 mL* |
| 1 lb. | *boneless veal, cut into ½-in. (13-mm) cubes* | *500 g* |
| 2 c. | *green apple, coarsely chopped* | *500 mL* |
| 1 c. | *onion, finely chopped* | *250 mL* |
| ½ c. | *sweet red pepper, cut into thin strips* | *125 mL* |
| 1 clove | *garlic, minced* | *1 clove* |
| 2 T. | *curry powder* | *30 mL* |
| 1 t. | *ginger* | *5 mL* |
| 1 c. | *apple juice* | *250 mL* |
| ¾ c. | *chicken broth* | *190 mL* |
| 2 t. | *cornstarch* | *10 mL* |
| ¼ c. | *cold water* | *60 mL* |
| ⅔ c. | *regular rice, cooked without salt* | *165 mL* |
| ½ c. | *unsalted peanuts* | *125 mL* |
| ½ c. | *raisins* | *125 mL* |
| ½ c. | *green onion, sliced* | *125 mL* |

In a Dutch oven, heat 2 T. (30 mL) of the oil over medium-high heat. Add veal, half at a time and cook, turning occasionally, about 5 minutes or until brown. Remove. Heat remaining oil and add next 6 ingredients. Cook, stirring, 2 minutes or until onion is tender. Return veal to Dutch oven. Stir in juice and broth. Bring to a boil, reduce heat and simmer 20 minutes or until veal is tender. Mix the cornstarch and water. Add to veal mixture. Stirring constantly, bring to a boil and boil 1 minute. Serve over rice with peanuts, raisins and onion.

**Yield:** 4 servings
**Exchange, 1 serving:** 2 bread, 3 fruit, 1 vegetable, 3½ high-fat meat
**Calories, 1 serving:** 660

*"A Diet for the Young at Heart" by Mazola.*

## Spicy Scrambled Egg Enchiladas

| | | |
|---|---|---|
| 8-oz. can | tomato sauce | 230-g can |
| 4-oz. can | green chilies, diced and divided | 120-g can |
| ½ c. | Kretschmer regular wheat germ, divided | 125 mL |
| 2 T. | green onion, chopped | 30 mL |
| 1 T. | vegetable oil | 15 mL |
| 4 | eggs | 4 |
| ¼ t. | oregano, crushed | 1 mL |
| dash | salt | dash |
| ½ c. | Monterey Jack cheese, grated and divided | 125 mL |
| 4 | flour or corn tortillas | 4 |

Combine tomato sauce, half the chilies, 2 T. (30 mL) of the wheat germ and the green onion. Mix well. Heat oil in a skillet. Add eggs, remaining chilies and wheat germ, oregano and salt. Stir to combine, breaking up the eggs. Cook over medium-low heat for 2 to 2½ minutes until eggs are softly set. Stir in half the cheese. Remove from heat. Spread 2 T. (30 mL) of the sauce on a side of each tortilla. Divide egg mixture among tortillas and roll up. Place seam side down on ovenproof baking dish. Top with remaining sauce and cheese. Bake at 450 °F (230 °C) for 10 to 12 minutes until thoroughly heated.

**Yield:** 4 servings
**Exchange, 1 serving:** 1 bread, 2 medium-fat meat
**Calories, 1 serving:** 211

*With the courtesy of Kretschmer Wheat Germ/International Multifoods.*

## Peanut Pork Chops

Well, Joe, here are your pork chops! You're right—they have fiber and they are good, but as I told you, there are lots of calories in a single pork chop.

| | | |
|---|---|---|
| 1 | egg | 1 |
| ¼ c. | water | 60 mL |
| ½ c. | salted peanuts, finely ground | 125 mL |
| 4 | lean pork chops (4 per lb. or ½ kg) | 4 |

Beat egg with water. Place in a shallow bowl. Place peanuts in another shallow bowl or plastic bag (I use the blender to grind the peanuts). Remove and discard any excess fat from chops. Dip chops first into the egg, shaking off excess, then into the ground peanuts, covering each chop. Grill chops on a medium-high barbecue for 8 to 10 minutes on each side.

**Yield:** 4 servings
**Exchange, 1 serving:** 2 high-fat meat
**Calories, 1 serving:** 218

## Stuffed Green Peppers

| ½ c. | Stone-Buhr long-grain brown rice | 125 mL |
| ¼ t. | salt | 1 mL |
| 8 medium | green peppers | 8 medium |
| 1 lb. | ground beef chuck | 500 g |
| ⅓ c. | onion, minced | 90 mL |
| 8-oz. can | tomato sauce | 227-g can |
| 1 t. | salt | 5 mL |

Place rice in saucepan with 1½ c. (375 mL) water. Add salt and bring to a boil. Cover and simmer until rice is tender and until all the water has been absorbed, about 40 minutes. Cut off and reserve tops of green peppers; scoop out and discard seeds. Place peppers upright in a baking dish. Mix together beef, onion, tomato sauce, salt and cooked rice. Stuff green peppers and replace tops. Pour ½ c. (125 mL) water in bottom of baking dish and bake in a 350 °F (175 °C) oven for about 1 hour.

**Yield:** 8 servings
**Exchange, 1 serving:** 1 bread, 1 lean meat
**Calories, 1 serving:** 166

*With the compliments of Arnold Foods Company, Inc.*

## Barley Hash

We like this for a quick lunch or supper. It is also a good recipe to help you use leftover beef.

| 1½ c. | water | 375 mL |
| ¾ c. | quick-cooking barley | 190 mL |
| 2 t. | salt | 10 mL |
| ¼ lb. | beef roast, cooked and cut into small pieces | 120 g |
| ¼ c. | onion, finely chopped | 60 mL |
| ¼ c. | green pepper, finely chopped | 60 mL |
| 2 T. | water | 30 mL |
| | salt and pepper | |

Bring water to a boil; stir in the barley and salt. Reduce heat, cover and simmer for 10 to 12 minutes or until barley is tender; drain thoroughly. Meanwhile, combine beef, onion and green pepper in nonstick skillet over medium heat. Add the 2 T. (30 mL) water, cover and heat until vegetables are tender. Drain off any excess water. Add barley and heat thoroughly. Season with salt and pepper to taste.

**Yield:** 4 servings
**Exchange, 1 serving:** 2 bread, 1 lean meat
**Calories, 1 serving:** 194

## Beef with Vegetables

An Eastern dish made easy.

| | | |
|---|---|---|
| ½ lb. | round steak ½-in. (13-mm) thick | 250 g |
| 2 | yellow onions | 2 |
| 4 | tomatoes | 4 |
| 1 | green pepper | 1 |
| ¼ c. | water | 60 mL |
| 1 T. | soy sauce | 15 mL |
| 2 t. | cornstarch | 10 mL |
| ½ t. | salt | 2 mL |
| 3 T. | vegetable oil | 45 mL |
| 1 slice | ginger root | 1 slice |

Cut steak across the grain into ⅛-in. (3-mm)-thick and 2-in. (5-cm)-long strips. Slice onions, tomatoes and green pepper into ½-in. (1.3-cm) wedges. Combine water, soy sauce, cornstarch, salt and 1 t. (5 mL) of the oil. Stir to blend and set aside. Heat remaining oil in wok or skillet; add beef strips and the ginger root. Stir and cook until well-browned. Add onions and stir-fry 1 minute. Add pepper and stir-fry 1 minute longer. Stir in cornstarch mixture and cook until sauce is clear. Add tomatoes and heat slightly.

**Yield:** 4 servings
**Exchange, 1 serving:** 1 vegetable, 2 medium-fat meat, ½ fat
**Calories, 1 serving:** 202

## Beef with Cauliflower

| | | |
|---|---|---|
| ½ lb. | flank steak | 250 g |
| 1 t. | salt | 5 mL |
| 1 T. | cornstarch | 15 mL |
| 3 T. | soy sauce | 45 mL |
| 1 large | yellow onion | 1 large |
| 2 | carrots, peeled | 2 |
| ½ head | cauliflower, cleaned | ½ head |
| 4 T. | vegetable oil | 60 mL |
| 2 cloves | garlic, crushed | 2 cloves |
| ½ t. | sesame seeds | 2 mL |
| ½ c. | water | 125 mL |

Trim off any fat from the steak. Cut across grain into ⅛-in. (3-mm) strips. Put meat in a mixing bowl, add salt, 1 t. (5 mL) of the cornstarch and 2 t. (10 mL) of the soy sauce. Stir to marinate meat; set aside for 30 minutes, stirring occasionally. Meanwhile, cut onion in half lengthwise; lay cut side down and slice crosswise into ¼-in. (6-mm) slices. Place onions in a separate bowl. Cut carrots in half on a long diagonal; slice on the diagonal into ¼-in. (6-mm) slices. Put carrots in a separate bowl. Cut cauliflower on the diagonal into ¼-in. (6-mm) slices. Add to the carrots. Heat a wok or heavy pan on high heat with 2 T. (30 mL) of the oil. Add garlic and sesame seeds; cook 20 seconds. Add remaining oil, heat, add meat and stir-fry quickly until brown. Remove meat from wok; keep warm. Add ¼ c. (60 mL) of the water to the wok. Add onions, cook and stir 2 minutes. Add carrots and cauliflower. Stir to mix. Cover and cook just until cauliflower is crisp-tender, stirring occasionally. Combine remaining cornstarch, soy sauce and water in a bowl or jar. Shake or stir to completely blend. Add meat to wok, stir to mix. Push meat and vegetables up side of wok. Add cornstarch mixture, cook and stir until thickened. Mix with the meat and vegetables. Pour onto hot serving platter.

**Yield:** 4 servings
**Exchange, 1 serving:** ⅔ bread, 1 vegetable, 3 medium-fat meat
**Calories, 1 serving:** 328

## Shrimp & Broccoli Chinese Style

Make sure you do not overcook this dish. Chinese food should be crispy.

| | | |
|---|---|---|
| 10 oz. | shrimp, cleaned | 300 g |
| ¼ c. | vegetable oil | 60 mL |
| 1 clove | garlic | 1 clove |
| 2 c. | broccoli florets | 500 mL |
| ⅔ c. | water | 180 mL |
| 1 t. | salt | 5 mL |
| 2 c. | fresh or frozen peas | 500 mL |
| 1 T. | cornstarch | 15 mL |

Cut shrimp into ½-in. (13-mm) lengths. Heat oil in wok or skillet, add garlic and cook until transparent. Stir in the shrimp and cook just until their color changes. Remove shrimp from wok and keep hot. Add broccoli to wok and cook 1 minute. Carefully, add water and salt. Cover and bring water to the boiling point. Add peas, cook 5 minutes. Return shrimp to wok. Blend cornstarch with 2 T. (30 mL) cold water; add to pan. Simmer and stir until mixture thickens and is clear.

**Yield:** 4 servings
**Exchange, 1 serving:** ½ bread, 1 vegetable, 2 medium-fat meat
**Calories, 1 serving:** 217

## Festive Party Chicken

| | | |
|---|---|---|
| 12 6-oz. | chicken breasts | 12 180-g |
| 1½ qt. | long-grain rice, cooked | 1½ L |
| 1½ c. | golden raisins | 375 mL |
| 2¼ t. | salt | 11 mL |
| 4 5-oz. cans | La Choy chow mein noodles | 4 150-g cans |
| 6 T. | butter, melted | 90 mL |
| 7½ c. | pineapple tidbits in their juice | 1875 mL |
| 4 c. | mandarin oranges | 1 L |
| 1½ T. | lemon juice | 22 mL |
| 6 T. | cornstarch | 90 mL |
| 6 T. | La Choy soy sauce | 90 mL |
| 6 T. | butter, cut into bits | 90 mL |
| 2 8-oz. cans | La Choy water chestnuts, drained and sliced | 2 240-g cans |

Cut chicken breasts in half, remove bones and cut through thickest part of each piece to form a pocket. In a bowl, mix rice, raisins, salt and 3 c. (750 mL) of the chow mein noodles; stuff ½ c. (125 mL) of the mixture into each breast; fasten with toothpicks and tie with string. Place chicken in buttered shallow baking pans and brush with melted butter; bake at 350 °F (175 °C) for 30 minutes. In a heavy pan, drain juice from pineapple and oranges and blend with lemon juice, cornstarch and soy sauce. Cook over medium heat, stirring constantly until sauce is thick and transparent. Remove from heat and add butter, pineapple, oranges and water chestnuts; mix well. Spoon over chicken and cover with aluminum foil. Bake at 325 °F (165 °C) for 30 minutes longer or until chicken is tender. Remove toothpicks and string. Serve sauce over chicken with remaining noodles on the side.

**Yield:** 24 servings
**Exchange, 1 serving:** 1 bread, 3 lean meat
**Calories, 1 serving:** 220

*Adapted from La Choy Food Products recipes.*

## Sweet Chicken

The sweet touches of pineapple and cherries add flavor and fiber to this colorful entrée.

| | | |
|---|---|---|
| 2 T. | margarine | 30 mL |
| 4 4-oz. | chicken breasts, boned | 4 120-g |
| 16-oz. can | tart cherries | 454-g can |
| 8-oz. can | crushed pineapple in its own juice | 227-g can |
| ¼ c. | dry sherry | 60 mL |
| 2 T. | soy sauce | 30 mL |
| 1 clove | garlic, minced | 1 clove |

| 1 T. | ginger, chopped | 15 mL |
| 1 c. | celery, sliced | 250 mL |
| ½ c. | sweet red pepper, cut in chunks | 125 mL |
| 1 T. | cornstarch | 15 mL |
| ¼ c. | water | 60 mL |

Melt margarine in a skillet and brown chicken breasts. Drain juices from cherries and pineapple into a mixing bowl. Reserve the fruit and add sherry, soy sauce, garlic and ginger to the juices. Stir to blend. Pour juice mixture over chicken. Cover and simmer 30 minutes. Remove chicken to warm serving dish and keep hot. Combine cherries, pineapple, celery, and red pepper in the pan. Dissolve cornstarch in the water and stir into pan. Cook and stir until mixture thickens. Pour over chicken.

**Yield:** 4 servings
**Exchange, 1 serving:** 2 fruit, 1 high-fat meat
**Calories, 1 serving:** 188

## Crowned Chicken Breasts

One of my daughter Beth Ann's favorite entrées.

| 3 T. | margarine | 45 mL |
| 4, 4-oz. | chicken breasts, boned | 4, 120-g |
| 2 T. | celery, very finely chopped | 30 mL |
| 1 T. | onion, very finely chopped | 15 mL |
| 1 lb. | mushrooms | 500 g |
| 2 t. | flour | 10 mL |

Melt 1 T. (15 mL) of the margarine in a nonstick skillet. Curl or roll breasts and fasten with toothpicks or poultry pins. Over low heat, brown chicken breasts on all sides. Lift and place breasts, skin side up, in a 10-in. (25-cm) pie pan. Remove toothpicks or pins. In the same skillet, melt 1 T. (15 mL) of the margarine. Add celery and onion; cook and stir until onion is tender. Slice mushrooms in half (if mushrooms are large, slice into thirds). Add mushrooms to pan and continue cooking; occasionally flip with a spatula until mushrooms are partially tender. Remove celery, onion and mushrooms from pan and set aside. Melt remaining 1 T. (15 mL) margarine in the skillet and stir in the flour. Cook and stir until flour is brown. Add enough water to make a thin sauce. Return mushrooms to skillet and stir to mix. Pour mushroom sauce over chicken breasts. Cover with aluminum foil. Bake at 300 °F (150 °C) for 40 to 45 minutes.

**Yield:** 4 servings
**Exchange, 1 serving:** 2 high-fat meat
**Calories, 1 serving:** 205

## Bran Parmesan Chicken

| | | |
|---|---|---|
| 1½ c. | Kellogg's bran flakes cereal | 375 mL |
| 1 | egg | 1 |
| ¼ c. | milk | 60 mL |
| ¼ c. | all-purpose flour | 60 mL |
| dash | salt | dash |
| dash | pepper | dash |
| ¼ t. | ground sage | 1 mL |
| 3 T. | Parmesan cheese, grated | 45 mL |
| 1 lb. | chicken, cut in pieces | 500 g |
| 1 T. | margarine, melted | 15 mL |

Crush enough cereal to measure ¾ c. (190 mL) in a shallow dish. Lightly beat together the egg and milk. Add flour, salt, pepper, sage and cheese, stirring until smooth. Dip chicken pieces in the egg mixture. Coat with crushed cereal. Place in a single layer, skin side up, in greased or foil-lined, shallow baking pan. Drizzle with margarine. Bake, uncovered, at 350 °F (175 °C) for about 45 minutes or until tender, without turning chicken while baking.

**Yield:** 4 servings
**Exchange, 1 serving:** 1 bread, 3 lean meat, 1 fat
**Calories, 1 serving:** 272

*From Kellogg's Test Kitchens.*

## Crispy Wheat Germ Chicken

| | | |
|---|---|---|
| 1 c. | Kretschmer regular wheat germ | 250 mL |
| 1 t. | dried tarragon, crushed* | 5 mL |
| 1 t. | lemon rind, grated* | 5 mL |
| ¼ c. | milk | 60 mL |
| 3 lb. | broiler-fryer chicken, cut up and skinned | 1½ kg |

Combine wheat germ, tarragon and lemon rind in a shallow container. Stir well to blend. Pour milk into another shallow container. Dip chicken pieces in milk, then in wheat germ mixture, coating evenly. Place on foil-lined 15½ × 10½ × 1-in. (39 × 25 × 3-cm) jelly roll pan. Bake, uncovered, at 375 °F (190 °C) for 40 to 50 minutes until tender.
*One teaspoon crushed oregano and a dash of garlic powder may be used instead of the tarragon and lemon rind.

**Yield:** 4 servings
**Exchange, 1 serving:** 1 bread, 5 lean meat
**Calories, 1 serving:** 357

*With the courtesy of Kretschmer Wheat Germ/International Multifoods.*

## Scalloped Turkey & Cauliflower

| | | |
|---|---|---|
| 2 c. | *fresh cauliflower, broken into florets* | 500 mL |
| 1½ c. | *turkey stock* | 375 mL |
| 2 T. | *whole wheat flour* | 30 mL |
| 1 t. | *parsley flakes* | 5 mL |
| 2 t. | *onion flakes* | 10 mL |
| 1 t. | *salt* | 5 mL |
| ¼ t. | *black pepper* | 1 mL |
| ½ lb. | *turkey breast, cooked* | 250 g |

Cook cauliflower in boiling, salted water for 6 minutes or until almost tender. Drain. Combine stock, flour and seasonings in a small saucepan. Cook and stir until mixture is slightly thickened. Place turkey breast in a greased baking pan. Arrange cauliflower around turkey breast. Pour sauce over turkey and cauliflower. Bake in a 350 °F (175 °C) oven for 20 to 25 minutes or until heated through.

**Yield:** 4 servings
**Exchange, 1 serving:** 1 medium-fat meat, 1 vegetable
**Calories, 1 serving:** 112

## Turkey Divan

| | | |
|---|---|---|
| 10-oz. pkg. | *frozen broccoli spears* | 285-g pkg. |
| ½ lb. | *unsalted, cooked turkey breast, thickly sliced* | 250 g |
| 2 pkg. | *Estee low-sodium mushroom soup mix* | 2 pkg. |
| ½ c. | *skim milk* | 125 mL |
| ⅓ c. | *cheddar cheese, shredded* | 90 mL |

Cook broccoli until just tender as directed on package; drain. With stems towards the middle, arrange broccoli in a 1½-qt. (1½-L) casserole or round 9-in. (23-cm) baking dish. Place turkey slices in an even layer on top. Combine soup mix with ½ c. (125 mL) boiling water. Blend in milk and cheese. Pour sauce over turkey. Bake at 375 °F (190 °C) for 25 minutes or until sauce begins to bubble.

**Yield:** 4 servings
**Exchange, 1 serving:** 2½ lean meat, 1 vegetable
**Calories, 1 serving:** 140

*For you from The Estee Corporation.*

# Ham Corncake

| | | |
|---|---|---|
| 1 T. | margarine | 15 mL |
| ¼ c. | onion, chopped | 60 mL |
| ¼ c. | green pepper, chopped | 60 mL |
| 1¼ c. | Featherweight corn flour | 310 mL |
| ½ c. | Featherweight oat flour | 125 mL |
| 5 t. | Featherweight baking powder | 25 mL |
| 1 t. | salt | 5 mL |
| 1 | egg, beaten | 1 |
| 1 c. | milk | 250 mL |
| 3 T. | margarine, melted | 45 mL |
| 8-oz. can | Featherweight golden corn, drained | 227-g can |
| 16-oz. can | Featherweight ham, drained and chopped | 454-g can |
| | Cheese Sauce (recipe follows) | |

Melt 1 T. (15 mL) margarine in a saucepan. Add onion and green pepper; cook until tender. Set aside to cool. In a bowl, combine dry ingredients—corn flour, oat flour, baking powder and salt. In another bowl, beat together the egg, milk and 3 T. (45 mL) melted margarine; add to dry ingredients and mix well. Add cooked onion and green pepper, corn and ham; stir to mix. Turn into a greased 9 × 9 × 2-in. (23 × 23 × 5-cm) pan. Bake at 400 °F (200 °C) about 30 minutes or until lightly browned. Serve hot with Cheese Sauce.

**Yield:** 6 servings

**Exchange, 1 serving with Cheese Sauce:** 2 bread, 3 medium-fat meat

**Calories, 1 serving with Cheese Sauce:** 374

## CHEESE SAUCE

| | | |
|---|---|---|
| 2 T. | margarine | 30 mL |
| 1 T. | cornstarch | 15 mL |
| ¼ t. | Featherweight mustard | 1 mL |
| 1 c. | milk | 250 mL |
| ½ c. | Featherweight cheddar cheese, shredded | 125 mL |

Melt margarine in a saucepan. Blend in cornstarch. Remove from heat. Mix in mustard. Add milk gradually, stirring until smooth. Cook and stir over medium heat until mixture boils; boil 1 minute. Add cheese and stir until cheese melts. Serve hot.

**Yield:** 6, 2⅔-T or 40-mL servings

**Exchange, 1 serving:** 1 high-fat meat

**Calories, 1 serving:** 101

*Based on recipes from Featherweight Brand Foods.*

# Casseroles

## Fresh Potato-Carrot Casserole

| | | |
|---|---|---|
| 2 t. | margarine | 10 mL |
| 1 c. | Kellogg's bran flakes cereal | 250 mL |
| dash | ground thyme | dash |
| 1½ c. | potatoes, sliced | 375 mL |
| 1½ c. | carrots, sliced | 375 mL |
| 2 T. | margarine | 30 mL |
| 5 t. | all-purpose flour | 25 mL |
| ½ t. | salt | 2 mL |
| dash | pepper | dash |
| dash | dried rosemary | dash |
| 1 c. | milk | 250 mL |

Melt 2 t. (10 mL) margarine. Stir in ¾ c. (190 mL) of the cereal and the thyme. Set aside for the topping.

Place potatoes and carrots in medium saucepan with salted water to cover. Bring to boil. Boil, uncovered, for 5 minutes. Remove from heat. Drain. In a large saucepan, melt the margarine over low heat. Stir in flour, salt, pepper and rosemary. Add milk gradually, stirring until smooth. Increase heat to medium and cook, stirring constantly, until mixture boils and thickens. Remove from heat. Gently stir in potatoes, carrots and remaining ¼ c. (60 mL) of the cereal. Pour into a round 1½-qt. (1½-L) casserole. Sprinkle with the topping. Bake at 350 °F (175 °C) about 25 minutes or until vegetables are tender.

**Yield:** 6 servings
**Exchange, 1 serving:** 2 vegetable, 1 fat
**Calories, 1 serving:** 105

*From Kellogg's Test Kitchens.*

## Soybean Casserole

| | | |
|---|---|---|
| 1 c. | Stone-Buhr soybeans, soaked in water overnight | 250 mL |
| 2 T. | saltpork, diced | 30 mL |
| 1 c. | celery, sliced | 250 mL |
| 2 T. | onion, chopped | 30 mL |
| 1 T. | green pepper, sliced | 15 mL |
| 3 T. | Stone-Buhr all-purpose flour | 45 mL |
| 1 c. | 2% milk | 250 mL |
| ¼ t. | salt | 5 mL |
| ¼ c. | Stone-Buhr wheat germ | 60 mL |

Cook soybeans in pressure cooker at 15 pounds pressure until tender, about 30 minutes; drain. Brown the saltpork in a skillet. Add the celery, onion and green pepper and cook for about 5 minutes or until vegetables are tender. Add the flour and mix well. Gradually add the milk and salt, stirring until it reaches the boiling point. Stir in the soybeans and pour the mixture into a baking dish. Cover with wheat germ. Bake at 350 °F (175 °C) for 30 minutes or until the wheat germ is golden brown.

**Yield:** 6 servings
**Exchange, 1 serving:** 1 bread
**Calories, 1 serving:** 78

*With the compliments of Arnold Foods Company, Inc.*

## Herbed Spinach Pasta

| | | |
|---|---|---|
| ¼ c. | Kellogg's All-Bran cereal | 60 mL |
| ¼ c. | Parmesan cheese, grated | 60 mL |
| dash | black pepper | dash |
| ¼ t. | dried basil | 1 mL |
| ½ t. | oregano leaves | 2 mL |
| 1 t. | fresh parsley, snipped | 5 mL |
| 3½ c. | spinach pasta ribbons | 875 mL |
| 2 T. | margarine | 30 mL |

Crush cereal into crumbs. Stir in the cheese, pepper, basil, oregano and parsley. Set aside. Cook pasta ribbons according to package directions just until tender. Drain. Gently toss hot pasta with margarine. Add cereal mixture, tossing until well combined. Serve immediately.

**Yield:** 5 servings
**Exchange, 1 serving:** 2 bread, ½ lean meat, 1 fat
**Calories, 1 serving:** 210

*From Kellogg's Test Kitchens.*

## Soybeans & Millet Casserole

| | | |
|---|---|---|
| 1 c. | Stone-Buhr soybeans | 250 mL |
| 1 c. | Stone-Buhr millet | 250 mL |
| ½ c. | onions, chopped | 125 mL |
| ½ c. | green pepper, chopped | 125 mL |
| ¾ c. | mushrooms, chopped | 190 mL |
| 1 t. | vegetable oil | 5 mL |
| 2 | eggs, beaten | 2 |
| 2 T. | margarine | 30 mL |
| ¾ c. | tomato juice | 190 mL |
| 1 t. | fresh marjoram, chopped | 5 mL |
| ¼ c. | brown sugar replacement | 60 mL |
| | salt to taste | |

Cook soybeans and millet according to package directions. Set aside. Sauté onions, green peppers and mushrooms in the oil for 10 minutes. Mix in remaining ingredients. Bake in well-greased casserole at 325 °F (165 °C) for about 45 to 60 minutes.

**Yield:** 6 servings
**Exchange, 1 serving:** 1 bread, 1 medium-fat meat
**Calories, 1 serving:** 142

*With the compliments of Arnold Foods Company, Inc.*

## Golden Barley

You don't always have to serve potatoes. Try barley for a new side dish.

| | | |
|---|---|---|
| ½ c. | cheddar cheese soup | 125 mL |
| 2 T. | hot water | 30 mL |
| 1 T. | catsup | 15 mL |
| 1½ c. | barley, cooked | 375 mL |
| ¼ c. | fresh parsley, chopped | 60 mL |

Combine cheese soup, hot water and catsup in a mixing bowl. Stir to blend. Add barley and thoroughly mix. Spoon into a greased microwave baking dish. Cover tightly. Microwave on MEDIUM for 7 minutes. Turn dish and stir slightly. Return to microwave, cook 3 minutes more. Remove cover, garnish with parsley.

**Oven method:** Increase water to ¼ c. (60 mL). Combine as above. Spoon into a greased baking dish or casserole. Cover tightly. Bake at 350 °F (175 °C) for 25 to 30 minutes or until mixture is bubbly. Garnish with parsley.

**Yield:** 4 servings
**Exchange, 1 serving:** 1 bread
**Calories, 1 serving:** 69

## Savory Bran-Rice Pilaf

| | | |
|---|---|---|
| ½ c. | long-grain brown rice | 125 mL |
| 1 | chicken bouillon cube | 1 |
| ¼ c. | margarine | 60 mL |
| ¼ c. | onion, chopped | 60 mL |
| ½ c. | celery, chopped | 125 mL |
| ½ c. | mushrooms, sliced and drained | 125 mL |
| ¼ c. | water chestnuts, sliced | 60 mL |
| 1 c. | Kellogg's All-Bran cereal | 250 mL |
| ¼ t. | ground sage | 1 mL |
| ½ t. | dried basil | 2 mL |
| dash | pepper | dash |
| ½ c. | water | 125 mL |

Cook rice according to package directions, adding bouillon cube instead of the salt and butter called for in the directions. While rice is cooking, melt margarine in a large skillet. Stir in onion, celery, mushrooms and water chestnuts. Cook over medium heat, stirring occasionally, until celery is almost tender. Gently stir in the cooked rice, cereal, sage, basil, pepper and water. Cover and cook over very low heat about 15 minutes. Serve immediately.

**Yield:** 6 servings
**Exchange, 1 serving:** 1 bread, 1 vegetable, 2 fat
**Calories, 1 serving:** 185

*From Kellogg's Test Kitchens.*

## Easy Lentils

I like this side dish with hamburgers instead of french fries.

| | | |
|---|---|---|
| 1 slice | bacon | 1 slice |
| ⅓ c. | green onions, chopped | 90 mL |
| ¼ c. | celery, chopped | 60 mL |
| 1¼ c. | vegetable juice | 310 mL |
| ½ c. | lentils | 125 mL |

In a small saucepan, brown the bacon. Remove and set aside; crumble when cool. Add onions and celery to pan, cook slightly. Add vegetable juice. Bring to a boil and stir in the lentils. Cover and reduce heat. Cook until lentils are tender, but not mushy, and liquid has been absorbed, stirring occasionally. Add crumbled bacon.

**Yield:** 4 servings
**Exchange, 1 serving:** 1 bread
**Calories, 1 serving:** 68

## Eggplant Casserole

| | | |
|---|---|---|
| 1 c. | Stone-Buhr brown rice | 250 mL |
| 3 c. | water, salted and boiling | 750 mL |
| 4 c. | eggplant, cubed | 1 L |
| ½ c. | onion, chopped | 125 mL |
| 1 lb. | lean ground beef | 500 g |
| 1¾ c. | canned tomatoes, drained | 440 mL |
| ½ c. | white wine | 125 mL |
| 1 c. | Parmesan cheese, grated | 250 mL |
| 1½ t. | salt | 7 mL |
| ¼ t. | pepper | 1 mL |
| ½ t. | granulated sugar replacement | 2 mL |

Stir brown rice into 3 c. (750 mL) of the boiling water. Cover and cook about 35 minutes. Rice should be almost tender, but still slightly firm; drain rice well. Pour boiling salted water over eggplant; soak eggplant for 5 minutes. Drain eggplant. Brown onion and ground beef. Add tomatoes and wine; bring to boil and simmer 5 minutes. Add drained eggplant, rice and all remaining ingredients. Transfer to a 3-qt. (3-L) casserole. Cover and bake at 350 °F (175 °C) for 30 minutes. Remove cover; increase heat to 400 °F (200 °C) and bake 15 minutes or until golden brown on top.

**Yield:** 8 servings
**Exchange, 1 serving:** 1 bread, 2 medium-fat meat, 1 vegetable
**Calories, 1 serving:** 258

*With the compliments of Arnold Foods Company, Inc.*

## Bulgur Pilaf

| | | |
|---|---|---|
| 1 T. | margarine | 15 mL |
| 1 c. | bulgur wheat | 250 mL |
| 2 c. | beef broth, hot | 500 mL |
| ¼ c. | chive, chopped | 60 mL |
| 3 T. | sweet red pepper | 45 mL |
| 3 T. | fresh parsley, chopped | 45 mL |
| | salt and pepper to taste | |

Melt margarine in a medium saucepan. Add bulgur and sauté for 1 minute, stirring constantly. Add broth, chive and red pepper. Stir to mix. Simmer, covered, over low heat for 15 minutes or until broth is absorbed. Stir in parsley. Season with salt and pepper. Spoon into serving dish.

**Yield:** 4 servings
**Exchange, 1 serving:** 2 bread
**Calories, 1 serving:** 132

## Tamale Casserole

| | | |
|---|---|---|
| 1½ lbs. | *lean ground beef* | 750 g |
| 1 medium | *green pepper, chopped* | 1 medium |
| 1 large | *onion, chopped* | 1 large |
| 1-lb. can | *whole tomatoes, undrained* | 500-g can |
| 8-oz. can | *tomato sauce* | 240-g can |
| ¼ c. | *Kretschmer regular wheat germ* | 60 mL |
| 2 t. | *chili powder* | 10 mL |
| 1½ t. | *salt* | 7 mL |
| dash | *hot pepper sauce* | dash |
| 1 recipe | *Wheat Germ Corn Bread (page 112)* | 1 recipe |
| 1 c. | *sharp cheddar cheese, grated* | 250 mL |

Cook beef, green pepper and onion over medium heat until beef is lightly browned. Drain. Stir in tomatoes, tomato sauce, wheat germ, chili powder, salt and hot pepper sauce. Simmer while preparing the batter for Wheat Germ Corn Bread. Pour hot meat mixture into greased 3-qt. (3-L) casserole. Spread evenly with the batter. Bake at 400 °F (200 °C) for 25 to 30 minutes until corn bread is golden brown. Sprinkle with cheese. Bake for 2 to 3 minutes longer until cheese melts.

**Yield:** 8 servings

**Exchange with 1 serving corn bread:** 1 bread, 2½ medium-fat meat
**Calories with 1 serving corn bread:** 224

*With the courtesy of Kretschmer Wheat Germ/International Multifoods.*

## Chicken Corn Hot Dish

| | | |
|---|---|---|
| 1 T. | *butter* | 15 mL |
| 1 c. | *fresh mushrooms, sliced* | 250 mL |
| 1 T. | *flour* | 15 mL |
| 1 c. | *chicken broth* | 250 mL |
| 2 c. | *chicken, cooked and diced* | 500 mL |
| 2 c. | *whole kernel corn, cooked* | 500 mL |
| 2 c. | *elbow macaroni, cooked* | 500 mL |

Heat butter in large skillet; cook until lightly browned. Add mushrooms and sauté until tender. Remove mushrooms from skillet. Add flour to remaining butter in skillet and mix well. Stir in chicken broth and cook over low heat until mixture thickens, stirring constantly. Add chicken, corn and macaroni. Stir to completely blend. Cook and stir over low heat until mixture is thoroughly heated.

**Yield:** 6 servings

**Exchange, 1 serving:** 1 bread, 2 vegetable, 1 high-fat meat
**Calories, 1 serving:** 228

## Great Bean Casserole

A quick Saturday lunch to make ahead and have extra time while it's baking.

| | | |
|---|---|---|
| 2 c. | *Great Northern beans, cooked* | *500 mL* |
| 1 cube | *chicken bouillon* | *1 cube* |
| 1 c. | *boiling water* | *250 mL* |
| 1 t. | *cornstarch* | *5 mL* |
| 3 T. | *cold water* | *45 mL* |
| 1 c. | *broccoli stems, chopped* | *250 mL* |
| 3 T. | *onion, chopped* | *45 mL* |
| ½ lb. | *freshly ground pork, cooked* | *250 g* |
| 1 t. | *salt* | *5 mL* |

Place beans in 1½-qt. (1½ L) casserole. Dissolve bouillon cube in boiling water; pour over beans. Dissolve cornstarch in cold water; add to beans. Add broccoli, onion, pork and salt. Stir to completely mix. Cover tightly. Bake at 350 °F (175 °C) for 2 hours or until beans are completely tender, adding more water, if needed.

**Yield:** 4 servings
**Exchange, 1 serving:** 1 bread, 1 vegetable, 2 lean meat
**Calories,1 serving:** 220

## Great Spaghetti

First, everyone likes this side dish, and second, it is a great way to use up those leftover spaghetti noodles.

| | | |
|---|---|---|
| 2 | *tomatoes* | 2 |
| ¼ c. | *garlic chive, chopped* | *60 mL* |
| ¼ c. | *green pepper, chopped* | *60 mL* |
| 2 c. | *cooked spaghetti noodles* | *500 mL* |
| | *water* | |
| | *salt and pepper to taste* | |

Core the unpeeled tomatoes; chop or cut into small pieces. Place in a medium saucepan. Add chive, green pepper and a small amount of water. Cover and cook until tomatoes are tender. Add cooked spaghetti. Stir to completely coat spaghetti. Simmer over low heat until spaghetti is hot. Season with salt and pepper.

**Yield:** 4 servings
**Exchange, 1 serving:** 1 bread, 1 vegetable
**Calories, 1 serving:** 97

## Company Casserole

| | | |
|---|---|---|
| 2 T. | butter | 30 mL |
| ¼ c. | green pepper, chopped | 60 mL |
| 1 T. | flour | 15 mL |
| 1 t. | salt | 5 mL |
| dash | pepper | dash |
| ½ c. | 2% milk | 125 mL |
| 1 | egg, lightly beaten | 1 |
| ¼ c. | sour cream | 60 mL |
| ½ c. | low-cal mayonnaise | 125 mL |
| 14-oz. can | La Choy fancy mixed vegetables, rinsed and drained | 420-g can |
| 7-oz. can | tuna, drained and flaked | 210-g can |
| 2 | tomatoes, peeled and cut into wedges | 2 |
| ½ c. | La Choy chow mein noodles, crushed | 125 mL |

Melt butter in a saucepan; add green pepper and cook 2 minutes. Blend in flour, salt and pepper. Gradually add milk; cook, stirring, until slightly thickened. Blend together, egg, sour cream and mayonnaise; stir into sauce. Add vegetables and tuna. Turn into buttered 1-qt. (1-L.) casserole. Arrange tomato wedges on top. Sprinkle crushed noodles over tuna mixture. Bake at 375 °F (190 °C) for 25 minutes.

**Yield:** 5 servings
**Exchange, 1 serving:** 1 bread, 1 medium-fat meat, 1½ fat
**Calories, 1 serving:** 221

*Adapted from recipes of La Choy Food Products.*

## Vegetable Linguine

| | | |
|---|---|---|
| 12-oz. pkg. | enriched linquine | 360-g pkg. |
| 4 small | stalks broccoli, thinly sliced lengthwise | 4 small |
| 1 medium | butternut squash, thinly sliced | 1 medium |
| 1 large | carrot, shredded | 1 large |
| 1 T. | onion, chopped | 15 mL |
| 32-oz. jar | meatless spaghetti sauce | 900-g jar |
| ½ c. | Parmesan cheese, grated | 125 mL |
| ½ c. | bean sprouts | 125 mL |

Cook linguine as package directs for 7 minutes. Add vegetables; cook 5 minutes and drain. In a medium saucepan, simmer spaghetti sauce 5 minutes or until thoroughly heated. Place pasta and vegetables in a large bowl. Add sauce and cheese; toss well. Serve 6 equal portions topped with the bean sprouts.

**Yield:** 6 servings
**Exchange, 1 serving:** 3½ bread, 2 vegetable, 1 medium-fat meat
**Calories, 1 serving:** 382

## Vegetarian Supper Pie

| | | |
|---|---|---|
| 1 c. | soda cracker crumbs (about 26 crackers) | 250 mL |
| ¾ c. | Kretschmer regular wheat germ | 190 mL |
| ½ c. | margarine, melted | 125 mL |
| 1 lb. (about 2 medium) | zucchini, sliced | 500 g (about 2 medium) |
| 1 medium | onion, sliced | 1 medium |
| 1 t. | dried marjoram, crushed | 5 mL |
| ½ t. | salt | 2 mL |
| ¼ t. | pepper | 1 mL |
| ¼ t. | dried tarragon, crushed | 1 mL |
| 1 c. | Monterey Jack cheese, grated | 250 mL |
| ½ c. | Parmesan cheese, grated | 125 mL |
| 2 | eggs | 2 |
| ⅓ c. | nonfat milk | 90 mL |
| 1 medium | tomato, thinly sliced | 1 medium |

Combine cracker crumbs, ¼ c. (60 mL) of the wheat germ and 6 T. (90 mL) margarine in small bowl. Stir well. Press evenly on bottom and about 1 in. (2.5 cm) up sides of 9-in. (23-cm) springform pan or on bottom and sides of 9-in. (23-cm) pie pan. Bake at 400 °F (200 °C) for 7 to 9 minutes until very lightly browned. Remove from oven.

Sauté zucchini and onion in remaining 2 T. (30 mL) margarine until crisp-tender. Add seasonings to vegetable mixture; stir well. Place half the vegetables in the crumb crust. Sprinkle with 3 T. (45 mL) of the wheat germ. Top with ½ c. (125 mL) Monterey Jack, ½ c. (125 mL) Parmesan cheese, remaining vegetables, and 3 T. (45 mL) wheat germ. Beat together the eggs and milk; pour over vegetable mixture. Arrange tomato slices on top. Sprinkle with remaining cheese and wheat germ. Bake at 325 °F (165 °C) for 40 to 45 minutes until hot and bubbly. Let stand 5 minutes before cutting and serving.

**Yield:** 6 servings
**Exchange, 1 serving:** 1 bread, 1 low-fat milk, ½ medium-fat meat, 4 fat
**Calories, 1 serving:** 420

*With the courtesy of Kretschmer Wheat Germ/International Multifoods.*

# Quick Breads

## Apple Fruit Loaf

The real American aroma—apples and spices baking!

| | | |
|---|---|---|
| ¾ c. | granulated brown sugar replacement | 190 mL |
| ½ c. | vegetable oil | 125 mL |
| 2 T. | dry sherry | 30 mL |
| 2 t. | vanilla extract | 10 mL |
| 1 c. | raisins | 250 mL |
| 1 c. | dates, chopped | 250 mL |
| ½ c. | walnuts, chopped | 125 mL |
| 1½ c. | apples, cored but not peeled, shredded | 375 mL |
| 3 t. | baking soda | 15 mL |
| 2 c. | all-purpose flour | 500 mL |
| ½ t. | salt | 2 mL |
| ½ t. | ground or grated nutmeg | 2 mL |
| ¼ t. | ground cinnamon | 1 mL |
| 2 T. | water | 30 mL |

In a large mixing bowl, stir together sugar replacement, oil, sherry and vanilla. Add raisins, dates and walnuts. In a small bowl, mix shredded apples with baking soda and stir to completely blend. Add to raisin-date-walnut mixture. Set aside. Sift together the flour, salt, nutmeg and cinnamon. Add to fruit mixture. Add water and blend thoroughly. Pour into 2 well-greased and floured loaf pans. Bake at 350 °F (175 °C) for 1 hour or until toothpick inserted in middle comes out clean. Cool in pan for several minutes. Remove loaf to wire rack for final cooling.

**Yield:** 1 loaf or 16 servings
**Exchange, 1 serving:** 1 bread, 1 fat
**Calories, 1 serving:** 100

## Banana Whole Wheat Bread

An extra bonus in a loaf of whole wheat bread.

| | | |
|---|---|---|
| ⅓ c. | *margarine, melted* | *90 mL* |
| ¾ c. | *granulated sugar replacement* | *190 mL* |
| 2 | *eggs, slightly beaten* | *2* |
| 3 | *bananas, mashed* | *3* |
| 1 c. | *all-purpose flour* | *250 mL* |
| 1 t. | *salt* | *5 mL* |
| 2 t. | *baking soda* | *10 mL* |
| 1 c. | *whole wheat flour* | *250 mL* |
| ⅓ c. | *boiling water* | *90 mL* |

With an electric mixer, beat margarine, sugar replacement, eggs and banana until smooth. Sift together twice the all-purpose flour, salt and baking soda. Stir whole wheat flour into the all-purpose flour mixture. Add dry ingredients alternately with boiling water to the banana mixture (add extra water if mixture is too dry). Pour into well-greased loaf pan. Bake at 325 °F (165 °C) for 1 hour or until toothpick inserted in middle comes out clean. Cool slightly in pan. Remove to wire rack for final cooling.

**Yield:** 1 loaf or 16 slices
**Exchange, 1 slice:** 1 bread, 1 fat
**Calories, 1 slice:** 115

## Banana Loaf

| | | |
|---|---|---|
| 2 | *egg whites, lightly beaten* | 2 |
| 1 c. | *bananas, mashed* | *250 mL* |
| ¼ c. | *sugar* | *60 mL* |
| ¼ c. | *Mazola corn oil* | *60 mL* |
| 1 t. | *vanilla extract* | *5 mL* |
| 1½ c. | *all-purpose flour* | *375 mL* |
| ½ c. | *walnuts, chopped* | *125 mL* |
| ½ c. | *raisins* | *125 mL* |
| 1½ t. | *baking powder* | *7 mL* |

In a medium bowl, stir together egg whites, bananas, sugar, oil and vanilla. In a small bowl, stir together flour, walnuts, raisins and baking powder. Stir into banana mixture until well mixed. Turn into a greased and floured 8 × 4 × 2-in. (20 × 10 ×5-cm) loaf pan. Bake at 350 °F (175 °C) for 60 to 65 minutes or until done. Cool in pan 10 minutes. Remove from pan. Cool completely on wire rack.

**Yield:** 1 loaf (16 slices)
**Exchange, 1 slice:** 2 bread
**Calories, 1 slice:** 160

*A recipe from Mazola.*

## Banana Bran Bread

This bread slices best on the second day.

| | | |
|---|---|---|
| 2 c. | all-purpose flour | 500 mL |
| ¼ c. | granulated sugar replacement | 60 mL |
| 1 T. | baking powder | 15 mL |
| ¼ t. | salt | 1 mL |
| ½ c. | whole bran cereal | 125 mL |
| ½ c. | skim milk | 125 mL |
| 1 c. | ripe banana (about 3), mashed | 250 mL |
| ⅓ c. | Mazola corn oil | 90 mL |
| 1 | egg, lightly beaten | 1 |

In a small bowl, stir together flour, sugar replacement, baking powder and salt. In medium bowl, stir together cereal and milk. Let stand 1 to 2·minutes or until cereal softens. Stir in bananas, oil and egg until well mixed. Stir in flour mixture just until blended. Turn into a greased and floured 8 × 4 × 2-in. (20 × 10 × 5-cm) loaf pan. Bake at 350 °F (175 °C) for 1 hour or until cake tester inserted in middle comes out clean. Cool in pan 10 minutes. Remove from pan. Cool completely on wire rack.

**Yield:** 1 loaf
**Exchange, 1 slice:** 1 bread, 1 fat
**Calories, 1 slice:** 124

*Adapted from a recipe contributed by Mazola.*

## Wheat Germ Corn Bread

| | | |
|---|---|---|
| ¾ c. | Kretschmer wheat germ | 190 mL |
| ½ c. | yellow cornmeal | 125 mL |
| ¼ c. | all-purpose flour | 60 mL |
| 1½ t. | baking powder | 7 mL |
| ½ t. | salt | 2 mL |
| 1 | egg | 1 |
| 1 c. | nonfat plain yogurt | 250 mL |
| 2 T. | margarine, melted | 30 mL |

Combine wheat germ, cornmeal, flour, sugar, baking powder and salt on waxed paper. Stir well to blend. Beat egg. Add yogurt and margarine, beating until smooth. Stir blended dry ingredients into yogurt mixture. Spread batter in greased, square 8-in. (20-cm) pan. Bake at 400 °F (200 °C) for 18 to 20 minutes until wooden pick inserted in middle comes out clean.

**Yield:** 16 servings
**Exchange, 1 serving:** ½ bread
**Calories, 1 serving:** 39

*With the courtesy of Kretschmer Wheat Germ/International Multifoods.*

## Cinnamon Whole Wheat Nut Bread

| | | |
|---|---|---|
| 2 c. | whole wheat flour | 500 mL |
| 1 c. | buttermilk | 250 mL |
| ¾ c. | almonds, finely chopped | 190 mL |
| ¾ c. | granulated brown sugar replacement | 190 mL |
| 1 | egg, slightly beaten | 1 |
| 1¼ t. | baking soda | 6 mL |
| 1 t. | salt | 5 mL |
| 2 t. | ground cinnamon | 10 mL |

Combine flour, buttermilk, almonds, brown sugar replacement, egg, baking soda and salt in a large bowl. Stir just to moisten flour. Pour into well-greased loaf pan. Sprinkle top of batter with cinnamon and stir it in to a depth of ¼ in. (6 mm). Bake at 350 °F (175 °C) for 45 to 50 minutes or until toothpick inserted in middle comes out clean.
**Yield:** 1 loaf or 16 slices
**Exchange, 1 slice:** 1 bread
**Calories, 1 slice:** 69

## Apricot Nut Bread

| | | |
|---|---|---|
| 1¾ c. | all-purpose flour | 440 mL |
| 3 t. | baking powder | 15 mL |
| ½ t. | baking soda | 2 mL |
| ½ t. | salt | 2 mL |
| ½ c. | sugar | 125 mL |
| ¼ c. | margarine, softened | 60 mL |
| 16-oz. carton | sour cream | 230-g carton |
| 1 | egg | 1 |
| 1 c. | dried apricots, finely snipped | 250 mL |
| ¾ c. | Kretschmer wheat germ | 190 mL |
| ½ c. | almonds, slivered | 125 mL |

Combine flour, baking powder, baking soda and salt on waxed paper. Stir well to blend. Cream sugar and margarine thoroughly in a bowl. Beat in sour cream and egg. Add blended dry ingredients to creamed mixture. Mix well. Stir in apricots, wheat germ and almonds, blending well. Spread batter in 2 greased 7 × 3 × 2-in. (17 × 8 × 5-cm) loaf pans or 8-in. (20-cm) layer pans. Bake at 350 °F (175 °C) for 45 to 50 minutes. Cool in pan 5 to 10 minutes. Remove from pan. Cool on rack. Wrap in foil or plastic wrap and store overnight for easier slicing.
**Yield:** 2 loaves or 32 slices
**Exchange, 1 slice:** 1⅓ bread
**Calories, 1 slice:** 82

*Adapted from a Kretschmer wheat germ recipe of Kretschmer/International Multifoods.*

## Super Zucchini Bread

| | | |
|---|---|---|
| 3 c. | all-purpose flour | 750 mL |
| 1¼ c. | wheat germ | 310 mL |
| 3 t. | baking powder | 15 mL |
| 2 t. | ground cinnamon | 10 mL |
| 1 t. | salt | 5 mL |
| 2 | eggs | 2 |
| 1 c. | granulated sugar replacement | 250 mL |
| ⅔ c. | vegetable oil | 180 mL |
| 2 t. | vanilla extract | 10 mL |
| 3 c. | zucchini, coarsely grated | 750 mL |
| 1 c. | walnuts, chopped | 250 mL |

Combine flour, wheat germ, baking powder, cinnamon and salt on waxed paper. Stir well to blend. In a bowl, beat the eggs until light. Add sugar replacement, oil and vanilla to eggs and beat well. Stir in the zucchini. Add the blended dry ingredients to zucchini mixture and mix well. Stir in walnuts. Spread batter in 2 greased 8 × 4 × 2-in. (20 × 10 × 5-cm) loaf pans. Bake at 350 °F (175 °C) for 55 to 65 minutes or until wooden pick inserted in middle comes out clean. Cool in pan 5 to 10 minutes. Remove from pan. Cool on rack. Wrap loaves in foil or plastic wrap. Store overnight for easier slicing.
**Yield:** 2 loaves or 32 slices
**Exchange, 1 slice:** 1 bread, 1 fat
**Calories, 1 slice:** 122

## Spoon Bread

| | | |
|---|---|---|
| 2 c. | white cornmeal | 500 mL |
| 2 c. | boiling water | 500 mL |
| 1¼ c. | skim milk | 310 mL |
| 3 | egg yolks, beaten | 3 |
| 1 t. | salt | 5 mL |
| 3 | egg whites, stiffly beaten | 3 |

Sift cornmeal and slowly stir into boiling water in a saucepan. Continue cooking and stirring until mixture is smooth. Remove from heat. Add milk, egg yolks and salt. Stir to completely blend. Fold in egg whites. Pour into a well-greased baking dish. Bake at 350 °F (175 °C) for 45 minutes.
**Yield:** 8 servings
**Exchange, 1 serving:** 2 bread
**Calories, 1 serving:** 149

## Carrot Bread

| | | |
|---|---|---|
| 1 c. | whole wheat flour | 250 mL |
| 1 c. | all-purpose flour | 250 mL |
| ¼ c. | sugar | 60 mL |
| 2 t. | baking powder | 10 mL |
| 1½ t. | ground cinnamon | 7 mL |
| ½ t. | salt | 2 mL |
| 2 | eggs, lightly beaten | 2 |
| ½ c. | skim milk | 125 mL |
| ⅓ c. | Mazola corn oil | 90 mL |
| 1½ c. | carrots, coarsely shredded | 375 mL |
| ¼ c. | walnuts, chopped | 60 mL |
| ¼ c. | raisins | 60 mL |

In a large bowl, stir together the flours, sugar, baking powder, cinnamon and salt. In a small bowl, stir together eggs, milk and oil. Add to flour mixture, stirring just until moistened. Stir in carrots, walnuts and raisins. Turn into greased 8 × 4 × 2-in. (20 × 10 × 5-cm) loaf pan. Bake at 350 °F (175 °C) for 1 hour or until cake tester inserted in middle comes out clean. Cool in pan 10 minutes. Remove from pan. Cool on wire rack.
**Yield:** 1 loaf (16 slices)
**Exchange, 1 slice:** 2 bread
**Calories, 1 slice:** 140

*A recipe from Mazola.*

## Johnnycake

An old favorite.

| | | |
|---|---|---|
| 2 c. | all-purpose flour | 500 mL |
| 5 t. | baking powder | 25 mL |
| 1 t. | salt | 5 mL |
| 1 c. | yellow cornmeal | 250 mL |
| 3 | eggs, beaten | 3 |
| 1 c. | skim milk | 250 mL |
| ½ c. | dietetic maple syrup | 125 mL |
| ½ c. | vegetable shortening, melted | 125 mL |

Sift together the flour, baking powder and salt. Stir in cornmeal and mix thoroughly. Add eggs, milk, dietetic maple syrup and shortening. Stir just enough to moisten flour. Pour into well-greased 3-qt. (3-L) baking dish. Bake at 400 °F (200 °C) for 30 minutes.
**Yield:** 12 servings
**Exchange, 1 serving:** 2 bread
**Calories, 1 serving:** 139

## Irish Whole Wheat Soda Bread

This was the way my mother always made Irish soda bread.

| | | |
|---|---|---|
| 2 c. | all-purpose flour | 500 mL |
| 2 c. | whole wheat flour | 500 mL |
| 1 t. | salt | 5 mL |
| 1 T. | baking powder | 15 mL |
| 1 t. | baking soda | 5 mL |
| ¼ c. | butter | 60 mL |
| 1 | egg | 1 |
| 2 c. | buttermilk | 500 mL |

Combine in a large bowl, the flours, salt, baking powder and baking soda. Stir to mix thoroughly. Add butter and work with your hands or a pastry blender until the mixture crumbles. Beat egg slightly and mix with the buttermilk until well blended. Add buttermilk mixture to flour and stir until blended. Turn into 2 greased and floured 8-in. (20-cm) cake or pie pans. Bake at 375 °F (190 °C) for 35 to 45 minutes or until toothpick inserted in middle comes out clean. Serve hot or cold.

**Yield:** 2 loaves or 32 slices
**Exchange, 1 slice:** 1 bread
**Calories, 1 slice:** 73

## Peanut Butter Bread

| | | |
|---|---|---|
| 1½ c. | all-purpose flour | 375 mL |
| 1 T. | baking powder | 15 mL |
| ½ t. | salt | 2 mL |
| ½ c. | sugar | 125 mL |
| 2 c. | Kellogg's bran flakes | 500 mL |
| 1⅓ c. | 2% milk | 440 mL |
| ⅓ c. | peanut butter | 90 mL |
| 1 | egg | 1 |

Stir together flour, baking powder, salt and sugar. Set aside. Measure cereal and milk into large mixing bowl. Let stand 2 minutes or until cereal softens. Add peanut butter and egg. Beat well. Stir in flour mixture. Spread batter evenly in greased 9 × 5 × 3-in. (23 × 13 × 8-cm) loaf pan. Bake at 350 °F (175 °C) about 1 hour or until done. Cool 10 minutes before removing from pan. Cool completely before slicing.

**Yield:** 1 loaf, 15 slices
**Exchange, 1 slice:** 2 bread
**Calories, 1 slice:** 135

*From Kellogg's Test Kitchens.*

## Puff-Cut Biscuits

| | | |
|---|---|---|
| 2 c. | all-purpose flour | 500 mL |
| 3 t. | baking powder | 15 mL |
| ¾ t. | salt | 4 mL |
| ¼ c. | margarine, softened | 60 mL |
| ¾ c. | skim milk | 190 mL |

Pour flour into a bowl and add baking powder and salt; stir to blend. Using a fork, stir in margarine until mixture looks like coarse meal. Add milk. Stir with fork until all ingredients are moistened and mixture forms a ball. Turn out onto lightly floured board. Shape with hands into a 12-in. (30-cm)-long roll. Cut into 12 pieces. Place pieces, cut side down, on ungreased baking sheet; flatten, if desired. Bake at 450 °F (230 °C) for 12 to 15 minutes.

### CRANBERRY PUFF-CUT BISCUITS

| | | |
|---|---|---|
| ½ c. | fresh or frozen cranberries, coarsely chopped | 125 mL |
| ¼ c. | granulated sugar replacement | 60 mL |

Combine cranberries and granulated sugar replacement. Prepare Puff-Cut Biscuits as directed above, except reduce milk to ⅔ c. (180 mL). Add sugared cranberries to biscuit mixture after you add the margarine. Complete as the basic recipe directs.
**Yield:** 12 biscuits
**Exchange, 1 biscuit:** 1 bread, 1 fat
**Calories, 1 biscuit:** 112

## Rice Fritters

| | | |
|---|---|---|
| 2 c. | brown rice, cooked | 500 mL |
| 3 | eggs, beaten | 3 |
| ½ t. | vanilla extract | 2 mL |
| ½ t. | fresh lemon peel, finely grated | 2 mL |
| ⅓ c. | all-purpose flour | 90 mL |
| ⅓ c. | granulated sugar replacement | 90 mL |
| 1 T. | baking powder | 15 mL |
| ½ t. | salt | 2 mL |

With a wooden spoon, beat together rice, eggs, vanilla and lemon peel until thoroughly blended. Sift together the flour, sugar replacement, baking powder and salt. Stir thoroughly into the rice mixture. Drop by spoonfuls into deep fat heated to 365 °F (180 °C). Fry until golden brown, turning if necessary.
**Yield:** 18 fritters
**Exchange, 1 fritter:** ½ bread
**Calories, 1 fritter:** 41

## Crunchy Blueberry Muffins

| | | |
|---|---|---|
| 1¾ c. | all-purpose flour | 440 mL |
| 1 T. | orange rind, grated | 15 mL |
| 2½ t. | baking powder | 12 mL |
| 1 t. | salt | 5 mL |
| ¾ c. | fresh or frozen blueberries, rinsed and drained | 190 mL |
| ⅔ c. | skim milk | 180 mL |
| ¼ c. | orange juice | 60 mL |
| 1 | egg | 1 |
| 2 T. | vegetable oil | 30 mL |
| 2 T. | granulated sugar replacement | 30 mL |
| ¼ t. | ground or grated nutmeg | 1 mL |

Pour flour into a large bowl. Add orange rind, baking powder and salt. Stir well to blend. Stir in blueberries. In a small bowl, combine milk, orange juice, egg and oil. Beat slightly. Add liquid ingredients to dry ingredients all at once. Stir just enough to moisten dry ingredients. Spoon batter into greased or paper-lined muffin-pan cups until ⅔ full. Combine sugar replacement and nutmeg. Sprinkle on batter. Bake at 425 °F (220 °C) for 20 to 22 minutes.

### MUFFIN VARIATIONS

Prepare Crunchy Blueberry Muffins as directed above except make the following changes.

**Crunchy Pineapple Muffins:** Omit blueberries. Drain an 8-oz. can (240-g) crushed pineapple, saving the juice. Substitute ¼ c. (60 mL) pineapple juice for the orange juice. Add crushed pineapple to dry ingredients.

**Crunchy Orange Muffins:** Omit blueberries. Drain an 8-oz. (240-g) can mandarin orange sections; chop finely. Add chopped orange sections to ingredients.

**Yield:** 12 muffins
**Exchange, 1 muffin:** 1 bread
**Calories, 1 muffin:** 79

## Our Best Bran Muffins

| | | |
|---|---|---|
| 1¼ c. | all-purpose flour | 310 mL |
| 1 T. | baking powder | 15 mL |
| ¼ t. | salt | 1 mL |
| 2 T. | sugar | 30 mL |
| 1 c. | Kellogg's All-Bran or Bran Buds cereal | 250 mL |

| | | | |
|---|---|---|---|
| 1 | egg | 1 | |
| 3 T. | vegetable oil | 45 mL | |

Stir together flour, baking powder, salt and sugar. Set aside. Measure cereal and milk into large mixing bowl. Stir to combine. Let stand about 2 minutes or until cereal softens. Add egg and oil. Beat well. Add flour mixture, stirring only until combined. Portion batter evenly into 12 greased 2½-in. (6.4-cm) muffin-pan cups. Bake at 400 °F (200 °C) for 20 to 25 minutes or until lightly browned.

**Yield:** 12 muffins
**Exchange, 1 serving:** 1½ bread
**Calories, 1 serving:** 100

*From Kellogg's Test Kitchens.*

## Raisin Bran Muffins

| | | |
|---|---|---|
| 1 | egg, lightly beaten | 1 |
| 1 c. | skim milk | 250 mL |
| 2 T. | Mazola corn oil | 30 mL |
| 1 c. | whole bran cereal | 250 mL |
| 1 c. | all-purpose flour | 250 mL |
| 3 T. | sugar | 45 mL |
| 1 T. | baking powder | 15 mL |
| ¼ t. | salt | 1 mL |
| ½ c. | raisins | 125 mL |
| | Cinnamon Topping (recipe follows) | |

In a small bowl, stir together the egg, milk and oil. Stir in cereal. Let stand 1 to 2 minutes or until cereal softens. In a large bowl, stir together flour, sugar, baking powder and salt. Stir in cereal mixture just until blended. Stir in raisins. Spoon into 12 greased 2-in. (5-cm) muffin-pan cups. Sprinkle with the topping. Bake at 400 °F (200 °C) for 25 to 30 minutes or until lightly browned. Serve warm.

### CINNAMON TOPPING

| | | |
|---|---|---|
| 2 T. | brown sugar replacement | 30 mL |
| ½ t. | ground cinnamon | 2 mL |

In a small bowl, stir together the brown sugar replacement and cinnamon. Makes about ¼ c. (60 mL).

**Yield:** 12 muffins
**Exchange, 1 muffin:** 2 bread
**Calories, 1 muffin:** 150

*A recipe from Mazola.*

## Lemon-Orange Muffins

| | | |
|---|---|---|
| 1¼ c. | all-purpose flour | 310 mL |
| 2 t. | baking powder | 10 mL |
| ¼ t. | baking soda | 1 mL |
| ¼ t. | salt | 1 mL |
| ⅓ c. | sugar | 90 mL |
| 1 c. | All-Bran cereal | 250 mL |
| ⅔ c. | milk | 180 mL |
| ¼ c. | orange juice | 60 mL |
| 2 T. | lemon juice | 30 mL |
| 1 t. | lemon peel, grated | 5 mL |
| 1 | egg | 1 |
| ¼ c. | shortening | 60 mL |

Stir together flour, baking powder, soda, salt and sugar. Set aside. Measure cereal, milk, orange juice, lemon juice and grated peel into large mixing bowl. Stir to combine. Let stand about 2 minutes or until cereal softens. Add egg and shortening. Beat well. Add flour mixture, stirring only until combined. Portion batter evenly into 12 greased 2½-in. (6.4-cm) muffin-pan cups. Bake at 400 °F (200 °C) about 20 minutes or until lightly browned.

**Yield:** 12 muffins
**Exchange, 1 muffin:** 2 bread
**Calories, 1 muffin:** 135

*From Kellogg's Test Kitchens.*

## Popovers

| | | |
|---|---|---|
| ¾ c. | whole wheat flour | 190 mL |
| ¼ c. | Health Valley Sprouts 7 cereal or | 60 mL |
| | Health Valley sprouted baby cereal, finely ground | |
| 2 | eggs | 2 |
| 1 c. | milk | 250 mL |
| 1 T. | butter, melted and cooled | 15 mL |

Using a whisk, combine flour and cereal. In a separate bowl, beat eggs lightly, then add milk and butter. Mix well, then add flour-cereal mixture and stir until light and smooth. Spoon mixture into 6 buttered custard cups until about half full. Arrange cups on a large, flat baking pan and place pan in a cold oven. Set oven control at 400 °F (200 °C) and bake popovers for 50 minutes or until puffed and brown. Serve immediately.

**Yield:** 6 popovers
**Exchange, 1 popover:** 1 bread, ½ high-fat meat, ½ fat
**Calories, 1 popover:** 150

*From Health Valley Foods.*

# Yeast Breads

## Whole Wheat Pocket Bread

| | | |
|---|---|---|
| 2 pkg. | active dry yeast | 2 pkg. |
| 1¼ c. | warm water | 310 mL |
| 1 T. | sugar | 15 mL |
| ½ c. | Kretschmer regular wheat germ | 125 mL |
| 1½ t. | salt | 7 mL |
| 1½ t. | vegetable oil | 7 mL |
| 1½ c. | whole wheat flour | 375 mL |
| 1 c. | all-purpose flour | 250 mL |
| 1 T. | sesame seeds | 15 mL |

Combine yeast and water in large bowl. Stir to dissolve yeast. Stir in sugar. Let stand for 5 minutes. Add wheat germ, salt and oil to yeast mixture. Stir well to blend. Stir in whole wheat flour with a wooden spoon. Beat in all-purpose flour to make soft dough that leaves sides of bowl. (Add a small amount of water if dough is too stiff.) Turn out onto lightly floured, cloth-covered board. Knead about 10 minutes until dough is smooth and elastic. Cover dough and let rise in warm, draft-free place about 1 hour until doubled.

Punch dough down. Divide into 10 equal pieces. Shape each piece into a ball. Let stand, covered, for 5 minutes. Sprinkle each ball with sesame seeds and additional wheat germ, if desired, before rolling. Roll into 6-in. (15-cm) rounds. Place on greased baking sheets. Let rise, covered, about 20 minutes. Bake at 450 °F (230 °C) for 5 to 7 minutes until browned. Remove from baking sheet immediately. Cool on rack. Cut in half and fill with desired fillings.

*Note*: If rounds don't puff completely, split halves open with tip of sharp knife.

**Yield:** 10 rounds
**Exchange, 1 round:** 2 bread
**Calories, 1 round:** 138

*With the courtesy of Kretschmer Wheat Germ/International Multifoods.*

## High Protein Bread

| | | |
|---|---|---|
| 1 pkg. | dry yeast | 1 pkg. |
| ¼ c. | warm water | 60 mL |
| 5 c. | Stone-Buhr all-purpose flour | 1¼ L |
| ½ c. | dry milk | 125 mL |
| ⅓ c. | Stone-Buhr soy flour | 90 mL |
| ¼ c. | Stone-Buhr wheat germ | 60 mL |
| 3 T. | granulated sugar replacement | 45 mL |
| 1 T. | salt | 15 mL |
| 1 T. | vegetable oil | 15 mL |
| 1¾ c. | water | 440 mL |

Dissolve yeast in warm water. Combine dry ingredients in mixing bowl. Add dissolved yeast, oil and water, mixing well to blend. Knead dough until smooth and satiny. Place in well-greased bowl. Cover and allow to rise in a warm place for about 1½ hours. Punch down by plunging fist into the dough. Fold over edges of dough and turn it upside down. Cover and allow to rise again for 15 to 20 minutes. Shape into 2 loaves; place in greased 9 × 5-in. (33 × 13-cm) loaf pans. Cover and allow to stand about 1 hour in a warm place, or until dough rises and fills pans. Bake at 400 °F (200 °C) for 45 minutes or until done. Remove from pans and cool on wire rack.

**Yield:** 2 loaves or 32 slices
**Exchange, 1 slice:** 1 bread
**Calories, 1 slice:** 71

*Based on a recipe from Arnold Foods Company, Inc.*

## Barley Flake Bread

| | | |
|---|---|---|
| ¾ c. | boiling water | 90 mL |
| ½ c. | Stone-Buhr barley flakes, more for sprinkling pan | 125 mL |
| 3 T. | shortening | 45 mL |
| ¼ c. | light molasses | 60 mL |
| 2 t. | salt, more for sprinkling pan | 10 mL |
| 1 pkg. | dry yeast | 1 pkg. |
| ¼ c. | warm water | 60 mL |
| 1 | egg, beaten | 1 |
| 2¾ c. | sifted Stone-Buhr all-purpose flour | 690 mL |

Stir together boiling water, barley flakes, shortening, molasses and salt. Cool to lukewarm. Sprinkle yeast on the warm water and stir to dissolve. Add yeast, egg and 1¼ c. (310 mL) of the flour to the barley mixture. Beat with an electric mixer at medium speed for 2 minutes. With a spoon, beat and stir in remaining flour until batter is smooth.

Grease a 9 × 5-in. (33 × 13-cm) loaf pan and sprinkle lightly with barley flakes and salt. Spread batter in pan. With a floured hand, gently smooth top and shape the loaf. Cover and let rise until batter just reaches the top of the pan, about 1½ hours. Bake at 375 °F (190 °C) for 25 to 35 minutes or until done. Remove from pan and cool on rack before slicing.

**Yield:** 1 loaf or 16 slices
**Exchange, 1 slice:** 1 bread
**Calories, 1 slice:** 73

*Based on a recipe from Arnold Foods Company, Inc.*

## English Muffins

| | | |
|---|---|---|
| 6 c. | *all-purpose flour* | 1½ L |
| 1 T. | *granulated sugar replacement* | 15 mL |
| 1½ t. | *salt* | 7 mL |
| 2 c. | *milk* | 500 mL |
| ¼ c. | *margarine* | 60 mL |
| 1 pkg. | *active dry yeast* | 1 pkg. |
| ¼ c. | *warm water* | 60 mL |
| ¼ c. | *cornmeal, more for sprinkling* | 60 mL |
| | *vegetable oil* | |

Spoon flour into measuring cup and level off. Pour onto waxed paper. Combine 2 c. (500 mL) of the flour, sugar and salt in large bowl. Stir well to blend. Heat milk and margarine together until warm to the touch (not scalding). Sprinkle yeast into warm water. Stir until dissolved. Add milk and yeast to ingredients in bowl. Beat with electric mixer at medium speed for 2 minutes, scraping bowl occasionally. Add 1 c. (250 mL) more flour. Beat at high speed for 1 minute. With wooden spoon, gradually stir in just enough remaining flour to make a soft dough that leaves sides of bowl. Turn out onto floured board. Knead 5 to 10 minutes or until dough is smooth and elastic. Place in greased bowl, turning to coat all sides. Cover with plastic wrap. Let rise in warm place about 1 hour or until doubled.

Punch down. Divide dough in half. On a board sprinkled with cornmeal, roll each half until ½-in. (1.25-cm) thick. Cut dough with floured 3-in. (7-cm) cutter. Place about 2 in. (5 cm) apart on greased baking sheet that has been sprinkled with cornmeal. Brush tops lightly with oil. Sprinkle with cornmeal. Cover. Let rise about ½ hour until light. Place on greased griddle preheated to 300 °F (150 °C). Bake about 15 minutes on each side until well browned. Cool on rack. Split muffins in half with fork and toast before serving.

**Yield:** 1½ dozen muffins
**Exchange, 1 muffin:** 2 bread
**Calories, 1 muffin:** 140

## Bran Batter Rolls

| | | |
|---|---|---|
| 1 c. | Kellogg's All-Bran or Bran Buds cereal | 250 mL |
| 3 c. | all-purpose flour | 750 mL |
| 2 T. | sugar | 30 mL |
| 1½ t. | salt | 7 mL |
| 1 pkg. | active dry yeast | 1 pkg. |
| 1 c. | milk | 250 mL |
| ½ c. | water | 125 mL |
| 2 T. | margarine | 30 mL |
| 1 | egg, lightly beaten | 1 |
| | poppy seeds (optional) | |
| | sesame seeds (optional) | |

In the large bowl of your electric mixer, stir together the cereal, 1 c. (250 mL) of the flour, the sugar, salt and yeast. Set aside. In a small saucepan, heat milk, water and margarine until warm. Add to cereal mixture. Reserve 1 T. (15 mL) of the egg. Add remaining egg to cereal mixture. Beat 30 seconds at low speed of electric mixer, scraping bowl constantly. Beat 3 minutes at high speed. By hand, stir in remaining flour to make a stiff batter. (Add a small amount of extra water if dough is too stiff.) Cover dough loosely. Let rise in warm place until doubled. Stir down the batter. Portion batter evenly into 16 greased 2½-in. (6.4-cm) muffin-pan cups. Brush tops of rolls with reserved egg. Sprinkle with poppy or sesame seed, if desired. Bake at 400 °F (200 °C) for 18 to 20 minutes or until golden brown. Serve warm.

**Yield:** 16 rolls
**Exchange, 1 roll:** 1 bread, 1 fat
**Calories, 1 roll:** 115

*From Kellogg's Test Kitchens.*

## Caraway Rye Bran Bread

| | | |
|---|---|---|
| 1 pkg. | active dry yeast | 1 pkg. |
| ¼ c. | warm water | 60 mL |
| 2 T. | granulated sugar replacement | 30 mL |
| ¾ t. | salt | 4 mL |
| 1 t. | orange peel, grated | 5 mL |
| 1 t. | caraway seeds | 5 mL |
| 1 c. | buttermilk, at room temperature | 250 mL |
| 2 c. | Kellogg's bran flakes cereal | 500 mL |
| 1 c. | rye flour | 250 mL |
| 1½ c. | all-purpose flour | 375 mL |
| 1 T. | milk | 15 mL |

In a large mixing bowl, dissolve yeast in warm water. Stir in sugar replacement, salt, orange peel, caraway seeds and buttermilk. Stir in cereal and rye flour. Gradually mix in enough all-purpose flour to make a soft dough. Cover and let rest 15 minutes. On lightly floured surface, knead dough about 5 minutes or until smooth and elastic. Place in greased bowl, turning once to grease top. Cover loosely. Let rise in warm place until doubled.

Punch down the dough. Shape into a smooth, round ball. Sprinkle cornmeal lightly on a baking sheet or grease lightly. Place dough on baking sheet. Flatten slightly. Cut a large **X** across top of loaf with sharp knife. Cover and let rise in warm place until doubled. Brush loaf with milk. Bake at 350 °F (175 °C) about 35 minutes or until golden brown and loaf sounds hollow when tapped. Remove from baking sheet. Cool on wire rack.

**Yield:** 1 loaf, 16 slices
**Exchange, 1 slice:** 2 bread
**Calories, 1 slice:** 140

*Adapted from a recipe from Kellogg's Test Kitchens.*

## Whole Wheat Bran Bread

| | | |
|---|---|---|
| 1 c. | all-purpose flour | 250 mL |
| 1 c. | whole wheat flour | 250 mL |
| 1 c. | Kellogg's All-Bran or Bran Buds cereal | 250 mL |
| 1 t. | salt | 5 mL |
| 1 pkg. | active dry yeast | 1 pkg. |
| ¾ c. | milk | 190 mL |
| 2 T. | molasses | 30 mL |
| 3 T. | margarine | 45 mL |
| 1 | egg | 1 |

Stir together the all-purpose flour and whole wheat flour. In the large bowl of your electric mixer, combine ½ c. (125 mL) of the flour mixture, the cereal, salt and yeast. Set aside. In a small saucepan, heat milk, molasses and margarine until very warm. Gradually add to cereal mixture and beat for 2 minutes at medium speed with electric mixer, scraping bowl occasionally. Add egg and ¼ c. (60 mL) of the flour mixture. Beat 2 minutes at high speed. By hand, stir in enough remaining flour mixture to make a stiff dough. On lightly floured surface, knead dough about 5 minutes or until smooth and elastic. Place in greased bowl, turning once to grease top. Cover loosely. Let rise in warm place until doubled.

Punch down dough. Shape into a loaf. Place in greased 8 × 4 × 2-in. (20 × 10 × 5-cm) loaf pan. Cover and let rise in warm place until doubled. Bake at 375 °F (190 °C) about 25 minutes or until golden brown.

**Yield:** 1 loaf, 14 slices
**Exchange, 1 serving:** 1 bread, 1 fat
**Calories, 1 serving:** 115

*From Kellogg's Test Kitchens.*

## Two-Tone Bread

| 2 pkg. | dry yeast | 2 pkg. |
|---|---|---|
| ½ c. | warm water | 125 mL |
| ¼ c. | granulated sugar replacement | 60 mL |
| ⅓ c. | vegetable shortening, melted | 90 mL |
| 1 T. | salt | 15 mL |
| 2½ c. | 2% milk, scalded and cooled | 625 mL |
| 5¼ c. | sifted Stone-Buhr all-purpose flour | 1310 mL |
| 3 T. | dark molasses | 45 mL |
| 2¼ c. | Stone-Buhr whole wheat flour | 560 mL |

Dissolve yeast in warm water. Add the granulated sugar replacement, shortening, salt and milk. Mix until sugar replacement and salt are dissolved. Add about 3 c. (750 mL) of the all-purpose flour and beat well, about 5 minutes. Divide dough in half. To one half, stir in enough of the remaining all-purpose flour to make a moderately stiff dough. Turn onto lightly floured surface and knead until smooth and elastic, about 5 to 6 minutes. Place in well-greased bowl, turning once to grease surface; set aside.

To the remaining dough, stir in the molasses and whole wheat flour. Turn onto lightly floured surface. Knead until smooth and elastic, about 5 to 8 minutes, kneading in an additional 3 T. (45 mL) all-purpose flour to form a moderately stiff dough. Place in well-greased bowl, turning once to grease surface. Cover both doughs and let rise until doubled, about 1 to 1½ hours. Punch down. Cover and rest on lightly floured surface for 10 minutes. Separately, roll out half the light dough and half the dark, each to a 12 × 8-in. (30.5 × 20-cm) rectangle.

Place dark dough on top of light; beginning at short side roll up tightly. Repeat with remaining doughs. Place in 2 greased 9 × 5-in. (23 × 13-cm) loaf pans. Cover and let rise until doubled, about 45 to 60 minutes. Bake at 375 °F (175 °C) for 30 to 35 minutes or until done. Remove from pans and cool on wire rack.

**Yield:** 2 loaves or 32 slices
**Exchange, 1 slice:** 1 bread
**Calories, 1 slice:** 69

*Based on a recipe from Arnold Foods Company, Inc.*

## No-Knead Whole Wheat Bread

| 3 c. | whole wheat flour | 750 mL |
|---|---|---|
| 1½ c. | uncooked quick-cooking or old-fashioned oats | 375 mL |
| 2 pkg. | active dry yeast | 2 pkg. |
| 1 T. | salt | 15 mL |
| 2½ c. | buttermilk | 625 mL |
| ½ c. | molasses | 125 mL |

| ⅓ c. | margarine | 90 mL |
| 2 | eggs | 2 |
| 2½ c. | all-purpose flour | 625 mL |
| | vegetable oil | |

Measure whole wheat flour into a large bowl. Add oats, undissolved yeast and salt. In a saucepan, heat buttermilk, molasses and the margarine together until warm to the touch. Add warm liquid and eggs to ingredients in the bowl. Blend with electric mixer at low speed until well mixed, about 30 seconds. Beat at high speed for 3 minutes, scraping bowl occasionally. Stir in all-purpose flour with a wooden spoon. Cover and let rise in warm, draft-free place about 1 hour or until doubled. Punch down. Place in 2 greased 2-qt. (2-L) casseroles or ovenproof bowls. Brush dough lightly with oil. If crust browns too quickly, cover loosely with foil during last 5 to 10 minutes. Remove from pans immediately. Cool on rack.

**Yield:** 2 loaves or 40 servings
**Exchange, 1 serving:** 1 bread
**Calories, 1 serving:** 73

## Herb Corn Bread

A batter bread—good for one of your bread exchanges.

| 1 pkg. | active dry yeast | 1 pkg. |
| ½ c. | warm water | 125 mL |
| 2 t. | celery seeds | 10 mL |
| 2 t. | ground sage | 10 mL |
| dash | ground ginger | dash |
| 13-oz. can | evaporated skim milk | 390-g can |
| 1 t. | salt | 5 mL |
| 2 T. | vegetable oil | 30 mL |
| 4 c. | all-purpose flour | 1 L |
| ½ c. | yellow cornmeal | 125 mL |

Dissolve yeast in water in a large mixer bowl. Blend in celery seeds, sage and ginger. Allow to stand at room temperature until mixture is bubbly. Stir in milk, salt and oil. On low speed, beat in flour, 1 c. (250 mL) at a time. Beat well after each addition. When mixture becomes too thick to beat with the mixer, stir in remaining flour and cornmeal with a spoon (dough should be heavy.) Divide dough and place into 2 well-greased 1-lb (500-g) coffee cans. (Dough may be frozen at this time for later use.) Cover and allow to rise until dough rises to top of can. Bake at 350 °F (175 °C) for 45 minutes. Serve warm.

**Yield:** 2 loaves or 28 servings
**Exchange, 1 serving:** 1 bread
**Calories, 1 serving:** 70

## Wheat Germ Croissants

| | | |
|---|---|---|
| 3 c. | all-purpose flour | 750 mL |
| 1¼ c. | butter, softened | 310 mL |
| 2 pkg. | active dry yeast | 2 pkg. |
| 1 c. | warm water | 250 mL |
| ¾ c. | Kretschmer regular wheat germ | 190 mL |
| 1 | egg | 1 |
| ¼ c. | sugar | 60 mL |
| ¾ t. | salt | 7 mL |
| 1 | egg | 1 |
| 1 T. | water | 15 mL |

Beat ⅓ c. (90 mL) flour and butter together until well blended. Spread into a 12 × 6-in. (30.5 × 15-cm) rectangle on waxed paper or foil. Refrigerate until firm, about 30 minutes. Dissolve yeast in warm water in large bowl. Add 2 c. (500 mL) flour, wheat germ, 1 egg, sugar and salt to dissolved yeast. Beat with electric mixer at medium speed for 1 minute. Gradually stir in remaining flour with wooden spoon to make a soft dough that leaves sides of bowl. (Add a small amount of extra water if dough is too stiff.) Turn out onto floured board. Knead 5 to 8 minutes until dough is smooth and elastic. Roll dough into a 14-in. (35-cm) square. Place refrigerated butter mixture on one side of rectangle. Fold dough over butter and pinch edges to seal. Roll into a 20 × 14-in. (51 × 35-cm) rectangle. Fold dough in thirds. Place on baking sheet. Refrigerate dough 10 minutes to firm the butter. Repeat rolling, folding and refrigerating the dough 3 more times. If butter begins to break through, sprinkle with flour to seal. Wrap and refrigerate dough for 2 to 3 hours after last folding.

Cut dough into thirds. Roll out each third separately and refrigerate remaining sections until ready to use. Roll the third of dough into a 20 × 14-in. (51 × 35-cm) rectangle. Cut crosswise into 4 equal pieces. Cut each piece diagonally to form 2 triangles. Roll up each triangle loosely, starting at 5-in. (13-cm) side and rolling towards the point. Place on ungreased baking sheets. Curve the dough rolls to form crescents. Cover loosely with plastic wrap. Let rise in warm draft-free place for 30 to 45 minutes until doubled. Brush dough with 1 egg, beaten with 1 T. water, just before baking. Bake at 350 °F (175 °C) for 18 to 22 minutes until golden. Serve warm, if desired.

**Yield:** 2 dozen croissants
**Exchange, 1 croissant:** 1 bread
**Calories, 1 croissant:** 70

*With the courtesy of Kretschmer Wheat Germ/International Multifoods.*

## Granary Beer Bread

| | | |
|---|---|---|
| 2 pkg. | active dry yeast | 2 pkg. |
| ½ c. | warm water | 125 mL |
| 1 c. | dark or regular beer, at room temperature (without foam) | 250 mL |
| 1 | egg, lightly beaten | 1 |
| 2 T. | brown sugar replacement | 30 mL |
| 3 T. | margarine, melted | 45 mL |
| 1½ t. | salt | 7 mL |
| 2 c. | stone-ground whole wheat flour | 500 mL |
| 1 c. | wheat germ | 250 mL |
| 1½ c. | all-purpose flour | 375 mL |
| 1 T. | vegetable oil | 15 mL |
| 1 | egg | 1 |
| 1 T. | water | 15 mL |

Dissolve yeast in warm water in a large bowl. Add beer, egg, sugar replacement, margarine and salt. Stir well to blend. Stir in whole wheat flour and wheat germ with a wooden spoon. Gradually stir in the all-purpose flour to make a soft dough that will leave the sides of the bowl. (Add a small amount of water if dough is too stiff.) Turn out onto floured board. Knead 5 to 10 minutes or until dough is smooth and elastic. Place dough in large, greased bowl, turning to coat all sides. Cover and allow to rise in a warm, draft-free place for 1½ to 2 hours or until doubled.

Punch dough down. Divide dough into 3 equal pieces. Shape each piece into a 16-in. (40-cm) rope. Braid ropes together. Shape into a ring and seal ends. Place in greased 9-in. (23-cm) springform or layer pan. Brush dough lightly with oil. Cover pan loosely with plastic wrap. Let rise for 1½ hours or until doubled. Brush dough with 1 egg beaten with 1 T. (15 mL) water. Bake at 350 °F (175 °C) for 40 to 50 minutes or until done. If crust browns too quickly, cover loosely with foil during the last 5 to 10 minutes. Remove from pan immediately. Cool on rack.

**Yield:** 1 loaf or 24 servings
**Exchange, 1 serving:** 1 bread
**Calories, 1 serving:** 78

# Desserts

## Wheat 'n' Oats Fruit Cobbler

| | | |
|---|---|---|
| 16-oz. can | pitted tart cherries | 480-g can |
| ¼ c. | granulated sugar replacement | 60 mL |
| 2 T. | cornstarch | 30 mL |
| 5 drops | red food coloring (optional) | 5 drops |
| 2 c. | fresh or frozen blueberries, rinsed and drained | 500 mL |
| ½ t. | almond extract | 2 mL |
| 1 c. | graham flour | 250 mL |
| 3 T. | granulated sugar replacement | 45 mL |
| 1½ t. | baking powder | 7 mL |
| ½ t. | salt | 2 mL |
| ¼ c. | margarine | 60 mL |
| ½ c. | quick-cooking or old-fashioned oatmeal | 125 mL |
| ⅓ c. | skim milk | 90 mL |
| 1 | egg, lightly beaten | 1 |

Drain cherries and save the liquid. Add enough water to make 1 c. (250 mL). Combine ¼ c. (60 mL) sugar replacement and cornstarch in a medium saucepan. Add cherry liquid, cherries and food coloring, if using. Stir to blend. Cook over medium heat until mixture comes to a boil. Reduce heat. Cook 1 minute, stirring constantly, until mixture thickens and is clear. Remove from heat. Add blueberries and almond extract. Pour mixture into 2-qt. (2-L) casserole. Set aside while preparing topping.

Measure flour into a bowl. Add 3 T. (45 mL) sugar replacement, baking powder and salt to flour. Stir well to blend. Cut in the margarine until mixture looks like coarse meal. Stir in oats. Add milk and egg. Stir just to moisten dry ingredients. Drop dough by spoonfuls onto warm fruit. Spread carefully to cover top. Bake at 400 °F (200 °C) for 25 to 30 minutes. Serve warm.

**Yield:** 8 servings
**Exchange, 1 serving:** 1 bread, 2 fruit, 1½ fat
**Calories, 1 serving:** 173

# Blueberry Basket Pie

| | | |
|---|---|---|
| 2 c. | all-purpose flour | 500 mL |
| 1 t. | salt | 5 mL |
| ¾ c. | vegetable shortening | 190 mL |
| 4–5 T. | cold water | 60–75 mL |
| 1 T. | lemon juice | 15 mL |
| 1 T. | margarine | 15 mL |
| | Blueberry Filling (recipe follows) | |

Measure flour into a bowl and add salt. Stir to blend. With a pastry blender, cut in half the shortening until mixture looks like coarse meal; then cut in remaining shortening until particles are the size of small peas. Add water a little at a time, mixing lightly with a fork. Shape dough into a firm ball with your hands. Divide dough in half. Flatten with the palm of your hand. Refrigerate, if desired, for easier handling and to prevent shrinkage.

Roll out half the pastry into a 12-in. (30.5-cm) circle on a lightly floured cloth-covered board. Place loosely in 9-in. (23-cm) pie pan. Fill with Blueberry Filling. Sprinkle with lemon juice. Dot with the margarine. Using a pastry wheel or sharp knife to make the lattice top, roll out remaining pastry and cut into ½-in. (13-mm) strips. Moisten rim of bottom pastry with water. Arrange pastry strips lattice-fashion over top of filling. Trim strips at edge of pan. Press firmly to lower pastry to seal. Fold lower pastry up over strips. Press firmly all around edge to seal tightly. Flute edge. Bake at 425 °F (220 °C) for 35 to 40 minutes. To prevent excessive browning of the crust, place a strip of foil around the crust edge. Remove for the last 15 minutes of baking.

## BLUEBERRY FILLING

| | | |
|---|---|---|
| ¼ c. | granulated sugar replacement | 60 mL |
| ¼ c. | all-purpose flour | 60 mL |
| ¼ t. | ground cinnamon | 1 mL |
| dash | salt | dash |
| 7 c. | frozen or fresh blueberries | ¾ L |

Combine sugar replacement, flour, cinnamon and salt in a large bowl. Add blueberries. Toss to coat evenly.

**Yield:** 8 servings
**Exchange, 1 serving:** 2 bread, 2 fruit, 3 fat
**Calories, 1 serving:** 365

## Fresh Apple Tarts

|          | Margarine Pastry (recipe follows)                          |          |
| -------- | ---------------------------------------------------------- | -------- |
| 3 large  | tart apples, peeled, cored, paper-thinly sliced            | 3 large  |
| 3 T.     | Mazola regular or unsalted margarine, melted               | 45 mL    |
| 1 T.     | brown sugar                                                | 15 mL    |
| ¼ t.     | ground cinnamon                                            | 1 mL     |
| 2 T.     | confectioners' sugar                                       | 30 mL    |

Divide Margarine Pastry into eight sections. Between 2 sheets waxed paper, roll each pastry section into a 5½-in. (14-cm) circle. Place on cookie sheets. Slightly flute edge. Top each pastry round with apple slices in overlapping rows. Stir together next 3 ingredients. With pastry brush coat apple slices with margarine mixture. Bake at 425 °F (220 °C) for 10 to 12 minutes or until golden brown. Sift confectioners' sugar over top. Broil 6 in. (15 cm) from heat for 1 minute or until bubbly. Serve warm.

### MARGARINE PASTRY

| 1¼ c.  | all-purpose flour                          | 310mL   |
| ------ | ------------------------------------------ | ------- |
| dash   | salt                                       | dash    |
| ½ c.   | Mazola regular or unsalted margarine       | 125 mL  |
| 2 T.   | cold water                                 | 30 mL   |

Mix the flour and salt. With pastry blender or 2 knives, cut in the margarine until fine crumbs form. Sprinkle cold water over mixture while tossing with the fork to blend well. Press dough firmly into a ball with your hands.

**Yield:** 8 tarts
**Exchange, 1 tart:** 2 bread, 1 fat
**Calories, 1 tart:** 158

*"A Diet For the Young at Heart" by Mazola.*

## Prune Casserole

A sweet ending to any meal.

| 4 c.   | whole wheat bread cubes, toasted      | 1 L     |
| ------ | ------------------------------------- | ------- |
| 2 c.   | prunes, cooked, pitted and sliced     | 500 mL  |
| 1 c.   | apples, chopped                       | 250 mL  |
| ½ c.   | prune juice                           | 125 mL  |
| 1¼ c.  | water                                 | 310 mL  |
| ½ t.   | salt                                  | 2 mL    |
| ½ t.   | ground cinnamon                       | 2 mL    |
| 2 t.   | margarine                             | 10 mL   |

Place half of the toasted bread cubes in a well-greased 1½-qt. (1½-L) casserole. Spread the prunes in a layer over the bread cubes. Arrange the apples in a layer over the prunes, then layer the remaining bread cubes. Combine prune juice, water, salt, cinnamon and margarine in a saucepan. Bring to a boil; cook for 3 minutes. Pour over prune casserole. Cover. Bake at 375 °F (190 °C) for 1 hour.

**Yield:** 8 servings
**Exchange, 1 serving:** ¾ bread, 2 fruit
**Calories, 1 serving:** 137

## Quick Cranberry Cobbler

| | | |
|---|---|---|
| 1 | *thick-skinned orange* | 1 |
| 1 c. | *water* | 250 mL |
| ½ c. | *granulated sugar replacement* | 125 mL |
| 4 c. | *cranberries* | 1 L |
| 1 T. | *butter* | 15 mL |
| 1 pkg. (8) | *biscuits* | 1 pkg. (8) |

Grate the orange rind. Juice the orange. Combine orange juice, grated rind, water, sugar replacement, cranberries and butter in a saucepan. Bring to a boil and cook for 1 minute. Spoon cranberry sauce evenly among 8 well-greased baking dishes or into a well-greased casserole. Top the cranberry sauce with biscuits. Bake at 450 °F (230 °C) for 10 minutes, reduce heat and bake at 350 °F (175 °C) for 20 minutes longer.

**Yield:** 8 serving
**Exchange, 1 serving:** 1 bread, ¾ fruit
**Calories, 1 serving:** 98

## Ground Almond Cookies

| | | |
|---|---|---|
| 1¾ c. | *all-purpose flour* | 440 mL |
| ½ t. | *salt* | 2 mL |
| 1 c. | *margarine* | 250 mL |
| ⅓ c. | *granulated sugar replacement* | 90 mL |
| ¾ t. | *almond extract* | 4 mL |
| 1 c. | *blanched almonds, ground or very finely chopped* | 250 mL |
| ¼ c. | *Powdered Sugar Replacement (page 19)* | 60 mL |

Measure flour onto waxed paper. Add salt and stir to blend. Cream thoroughly the margarine, granulated sugar replacement and almond extract. Add blended dry ingredients and almonds to creamed mixture. Mix well. Shape dough into 1-in. (2.5-cm) balls or crescents. Place on ungreased baking sheets. Bake at 375 °F (190 °C) for 10 to 12 minutes until lightly browned. Remove from baking sheets. Cool slightly on rack. Roll in powdered sugar replacement. Cool.

**Yield:** 4 dozen cookies
**Exchange, 1 cookie:** ⅓ bread, 1 fat
**Calories, 1 cookie:** 60

## Sunflower Seed Cookies

| | | |
|---|---|---|
| 1 c. | margarine | 250 mL |
| ¾ c. | granulated brown sugar replacement | 190 mL |
| ½ c. | granulated sugar replacement | 125 mL |
| 2 | eggs | 2 |
| 1 t. | vanilla | 5 mL |
| 3 T. | water | 45 mL |
| 1½ c. | Stone-Buhr all-purpose flour | 375 mL |
| ¾ t. | salt | 4 mL |
| 1 t. | baking soda | 5 mL |
| 3 c. | Stone-Buhr quick-cooking rolled oats | 750 mL |
| 1 c. | Stone-Buhr sunflower seeds | 250 mL |

Thoroughly cream together the margarine and sugar replacements. Add eggs and vanilla and beat to blend well. Add water, flour, salt, soda and rolled oats. Mix thoroughly. (Add a small amount of extra water if dough is too stiff.) Gently blend in the sunflower seeds. Form dough into long rolls about 1½ in. (3.8 cm) in diameter. Wrap in clear plastic and chill thoroughly. Slice ¼-in. (6-mm) thick. Arrange on ungreased cookie sheet and bake at 350 °F (175 °C) for 8 to 10 minutes or until lightly browned. Cool on wire racks and store in airtight containers.
**Yield:** 9 dozen
**Exchange, 1 serving:** 1 bread
**Calories, 1 serving:** 64

*Based on a recipe with the compliments of Arnold Foods Company, Inc.*

## Fig Bars

| | | |
|---|---|---|
| 1½ c. | all-purpose flour | 375 mL |
| ¾ c. | Kretschmer wheat germ | 190 mL |
| ¼ c. | sugar | 60 mL |
| 1½ t. | orange rind, grated | 7 mL |
| ¼ t. | salt | 1 ml |
| ½ c. | margarine | 125 mL |
| ¾ c. | orange juice, divided | 190 mL |
| 8 oz. | moist-pack figs | 240 g |

Combine flour, ½ c. (125 mL) of the wheat germ, sugar, orange rind and salt in bowl. Stir well to blend. Cut in margarine with pastry blender until mixture looks like fine crumbs. Add ¼ c. (60 mL) of the orange juice, a little at a time, mixing lightly with fork. With your hands, shape into a firm ball. Trim stems from figs. Purée figs in blender container with remaining ½ c. (125 mL) orange juice for 30 seconds. Stir in remaining ¼ c. (60 mL) wheat germ.

Roll out dough into a 14 × 12-in. (35.6 × 30.5 cm) rectangle on a lightly floured cloth-covered board. Cut lengthwise into 3 4-in. (10-cm)-wide strips. Place on ungreased baking sheets. Spoon about ⅓ c. (90 mL) of the filling on each strip to within ½ in. (13 mm) of the long edges. Fold dough over to cover filling. Press long edges together with tines of fork. Bake at 350 °F (175 °C) for 17 to 20 minutes until golden. Remove from baking sheet. Cool on rack. Slice diagonally into 1-in. (2.5-cm)-wide strips.

**Yield:** 36 cookies

**Exchange, 1 cookie:** ½ bread, ⅓ fruit

**Calories, 1 cookie:** 45

*With the courtesy of Kretschmer Wheat Germ/International Multifoods.*

## Date Sandwich Bars

| 2 c. | pitted dates, snipped | 500 mL |
|---|---|---|
| 1 c. | water | 250 mL |
| 1 t. | orange rind, grated | 5 mL |
| 2 T. | orange juice | 30 mL |
| 1 t. | lemon juice | 5 mL |
| 1½ c. | all-purpose flour | 375 mL |
| 1½ c. | uncooked oatmeal | 375 mL |
| 2 T. | brown sugar replacement | 30 mL |
| 1 t. | baking powder | 5 mL |
| ½ t. | salt | 2 mL |
| ¾ c. | butter | 190 mL |

Combine dates, water, rind and juices in a saucepan. Blend well. Cook over low heat, stirring occasionally, until thickened, about 10 minutes. Cool while preparing crumb mixture. Measure flour into a large bowl. Add all remaining ingredients except butter. Stir well to blend. Cut in butter with pastry blender until particles are the size of small peas. Spread half of the crumb mixture in a greased 13 × 9 × 2-in. (33 × 23 × 5-cm) pan. Press down. Spread cooled date filling evenly over mixture in pan. Cover with remaining crumb mixture. Pat down lightly. Bake at 375 °F (190 °C) for 25 to 30 minutes until golden brown. Cool in pan on rack. Cut into bars.

**Yield:** 3 dozen bars

**Exchange, 1 bar:** 1½ fruit, 1 fat

**Calories, 1 bar:** 97

## Whole Wheat Oat Cookies

| | | |
|---|---|---|
| 1¼ c. | whole wheat flour | 310 mL |
| ½ t. | baking soda | 2 mL |
| ½ t. | salt | 2 mL |
| ½ t. | ground ginger | 2 mL |
| ½ t. | ground cinnamon | 2 mL |
| 1 | egg | 1 |
| ½ c. | Mazola corn oil | 125 mL |
| ⅓ c. | brown sugar replacement | 90 mL |
| ¼ c. | honey | 60 mL |
| 1 c. | quick-cooking oats | 250 mL |
| ½ c. | raisins | 125 mL |

In a small bowl, stir together flour, baking soda, salt, ginger and cinnamon. In a large bowl with mixer at medium speed, beat egg, oil, brown sugar replacement and honey until mixture is thick and smooth. Reduce speed to low. Add flour mixture; beat until blended. Stir in oats and raisins. Drop by heaping teaspoonfuls 2 in. (5 cm) apart onto greased cookie sheets. Bake in 375 °F (190 °C) oven 6 to 8 minutes or until edges are browned.

**Yield:** 4½ dozen
**Exchange, 2 cookies:** 1 bread
**Calories, 2 cookies:** 64

*Adapted from a special recipe from Mazola.*

## Coffee Coconut Cake

| | | |
|---|---|---|
| 1½ c. | all-purpose flour | 375 mL |
| 1 t. | baking soda | 5 mL |
| ½ t. | salt | 2 mL |
| 1 t. | ground cinnamon | 5 mL |
| ½ c. | granulated sugar replacement | 125 mL |
| ½ c. | Kellogg's All-Bran or Bran Buds cereal | 125 mL |
| 1 c. | cold strong coffee | 250 mL |
| ¼ c. | vegetable oil | 60 mL |
| 1 T. | vinegar | 15 mL |
| ½ t. | almond flavoring | 2 mL |
| ½ c. | flaked coconut | 125 mL |

Stir together flour, soda, salt, cinnamon and sugar replacement. Set aside. Measure cereal and coffee into a large bowl. Stir to combine. Let stand about 2 minutes or until cereal softens. Stir in oil, vinegar, almond flavoring and ⅓ c. (90 mL) of the coconut. Add flour mixture, mixing until well combined. Spread evenly in greased 8 × 8 × 2-in. (20

× 20 × 5-cm) baking pan. Sprinkle remaining coconut over batter. Bake at 350 °F (175 °C) about 25 minutes or until cake tests done. Serve warm or cool with whipped topping, if desired.

**Yield:** 12 servings

**Exchange, 1 serving:** (without whipped topping): 1 bread, 1 fat

**Calories, 1 serving:** (without whipped topping): 117

*From Kellogg's Test Kitchens.*

## Apple Crunch Cake

| | | |
|---|---|---|
| ⅓ c. | Kellogg's bran flakes cereal | 90 mL |
| 3 T. | granulated sugar replacement | 45 mL |
| ¼ t. | salt | 1 mL |
| ¼ t. | ground cinnamon | 1 mL |
| 3 T. | margarine | 45 mL |
| 1 c. | Kellogg's bran flakes cereal | 250 mL |
| 1¼ c. | all-purpose flour | 310 mL |
| 2 t. | baking powder | 10 mL |
| ½ t. | salt | 2 mL |
| ¼ c. | margarine, softened | 60 mL |
| ½ c. | granulated sugar replacement | 125 mL |
| 1 | egg | 1 |
| 1 t. | lemon peel, grated | 5 mL |
| ½ c. | skim milk | 125 mL |
| 2½ c. | pared apples, coarsely chopped | 625 mL |

Stir together first 4 ingredients. Cut in the 3 T. (45 mL) margarine until mixture is crumbly. Set aside to use as a topping. Crush the 1 c. (250 mL) cereal to ½ c. (125 mL). Stir in flour, baking powder and salt. Set aside.

In a large mixing bowl, beat margarine, sugar replacement, egg and lemon peel until light and fluffy. Add flour mixture alternately with milk, mixing well after each addition. Stir in apples. Spread evenly in greased 9 × 9 × 2-in. (23 × 23 × 5-cm) baking pan. Sprinkle evenly with cereal topping. Bake at 375 °F (190 °C) about 35 minutes or until cake tests done. Cool. Serve with nondairy whipped topping, if desired.

**Yield:** 16 servings

**Exchange, 1 serving:** (without whipped topping): 1 bread, 1 fat

**Calories, 1 serving:** (without whipped topping): 105

*Based on a recipe from Kellogg's Test Kitchens.*

## Wheat Germ Strawberry Shortcake

| | | |
|---|---|---|
| 1 c. | all-purpose flour | 250 mL |
| ¾ c. | wheat germ | 190 mL |
| ¼ c. | granulated sugar replacement | 60 mL |
| 1½ t. | baking powder | 7 mL |
| ¼ t. | salt | 1 mL |
| ¼ t. | ground cinnamon | 1 mL |
| ¼ c. | vegetable shortening | 60 mL |
| ⅓ c. | water | 90 mL |
| ¼ c. | margarine, melted | 60 mL |
| 2 t. | wheat germ | 10 mL |
| 1 qt. | fresh strawberries, sliced and sweetened | 1 L |
| 1 c. | nondairy whipped topping | 250 mL |

Combine flour, ¾ c. (190 mL) wheat germ, sugar replacement, baking powder, salt and cinnamon in a bowl. Stir well to blend. Cut in the shortening with pastry blender until mixture looks like coarse meal. Add water and margarine. Mix well. Divide dough in half. Spread each half into a 7-in. (18-cm) circle on a greased baking sheet. Sprinkle with the remaining 2 t. (10 mL) wheat germ. Bake at 400 °F (200 °C) for 12 to 15 minutes until lightly browned. Remove from baking sheet. Cool on a rack. Layer with strawberries and nondairy whipped topping.
**Yield:** 8 servings
**Exchange, 1 serving:** 2 bread, ½ fruit, 2 fat
**Calories, 1 serving:** 242

## Rice Pudding

| | | |
|---|---|---|
| 4 c. | water | 1 L |
| ¾ c. | Stone-Buhr long-grain brown rice | 190 mL |
| ½ c. | granulated sugar replacement | 125 mL |
| ¼ c. | golden raisins | 60 mL |
| ¼ c. | margarine | 60 mL |
| 3 in. | vanilla bean | 7 cm |
| 3 in. | cinnamon stick | 7 cm |
| 3 c. | skim milk | 750 mL |
| ½ c. | fresh apricots, chopped | 125 mL |
| 3 | eggs, separated | 3 |
| ¼ t. | cream of tartar | 1 mL |

Bring water to a boil. Add rice and boil for 20 minutes. Drain rice in a sieve. Place rice, sugar replacement, raisins, 2 T. (30 mL) of the margarine, vanilla bean, cinnamon stick and milk in a saucepan. Bring to a boil, cover and cook over low heat, stirring occasionally, for about 1¼ hours or until most of the milk is absorbed. Stir in remaining margarine. Spread out in a pan and cool. Remove the vanilla and cinnamon pieces from the rice and mix in apricots and egg yolks. In a bowl, beat the egg whites with the cream of tartar until soft peaks form. Fold gently into rice mixture. Pour into a mould and place in a pan of hot water. Bake at 325 °F (165 °C) for 1 hour. Remove from oven and let stand at room temperature for 1 hour before serving.

**Yield:** 8 servings

**Exchange, 1 serving:** 1½ fruit, ½ full-fat milk

**Calories, 1 serving:** 142

*Based on a recipe with the compliments of Arnold Foods Company, Inc.*

## Sweet Potato Pudding

A favorite at our home on holidays.

| | | |
|---|---|---|
| 4 | eggs | 4 |
| 2 c. | skim milk | 500 mL |
| 3 c. | sweet potatoes, peeled and grated | 750 mL |
| 3 T. | butter | 45 mL |
| 1¼ c. | granulated brown sugar replacement | 310 mL |
| ¼ c. | wheat germ | 60 mL |
| ½ t. | ground cinnamon | 2 mL |
| ¼ t. | ground cloves | 1 mL |
| ¼ t. | ground allspice | 1 mL |
| ¼ t. | salt | 1 mL |

Beat eggs until light and fluffy. Add remaining ingredients and stir to mix well. Pour into a well-greased baking dish. Bake at 325 °F (165 °C) for 30 minutes or until set and top is lightly browned.

**Yield:** 10 servings

**Exchange, 1 serving:** 1 bread, ½ high-fat meat

**Calories, 1 serving:** 129

## Flaming Peaches

A fast but exotic dessert.

| | | |
|---|---|---|
| 6 | canned peach halves in their own juice | 6 |
| ¼ c. | Raspberry Preserves (page 19) | 60 mL |
| ¼ c. | brandy | 60 mL |

Drain peach halves. Arrange in 6 shallow baking dishes. Melt preserves, stirring constantly. Brush peaches with preserves. Drizzle brandy over peaches; ignite. Serve immediately.

**Yield:** 6 servings

**Exchange, 1 serving:** 1 fruit

**Calories, 1 serving:** 30

## Apple Indian Pudding

| | | |
|---|---|---|
| 1 qt. | 2% milk | 1 L |
| ½ c. | cornmeal | 125 mL |
| ⅓ c. | liquid fructose | 90 mL |
| ⅓ c. | granulated brown sugar replacement | 90 mL |
| 1 t. | salt | 5 mL |
| 1 t. | ground cinnamon | 5 mL |
| ¼ t. | ground ginger | 1 mL |
| 2 | apples | 2 |
| 1 c. | skim milk | 250 mL |

Bring milk to a boil. Slowly stir in the cornmeal and cook until thickened. Remove from heat. Stir in fructose, sugar replacement, salt, cinnamon and ginger. Core and thinly slice the apples. Layer cornmeal mixture alternately with apple slices in well-greased casserole. Pour skim milk over entire mixture. Bake at 275 °F (135 °C) for 1 hour.
**Yield:** 10 servings
**Exchange, 1 serving:** 1 bread, ¾ fruit
**Calories, 1 serving:** 97

## Crepes

| | | |
|---|---|---|
| 2 | eggs | 2 |
| 2 T. | safflower oil | 30 mL |
| 2 c. | milk | 500 mL |
| 1 c. | Health Valley 7 sprouted grains pancake mix | 250 mL |
| | oil for cooking | |

In medium bowl, combine eggs, oil and milk. Mix well. Add pancake mix. Stir well. Lightly grease 8-in. (20-cm) skillet or omelet pan. Heat over medium-high heat. Add just enough batter to thinly cover the bottom. Cook until bubbles appear. Turn and cook other side. Remove crepe to warm platter. Repeat until batter is used up.
*Note*: Crepes may be made ahead of time and frozen. To freeze, put a piece of waxed paper between each 4 crepes for easier separation. When planning to use, thaw crepes overnight in refrigerator. To make crepes soft enough to roll, heat in 325 °F (165 °C) oven for 15 minutes.
**Yield:** 22 crepes
**Exchange, 1 crepe:** ¼ bread, ½ low-fat milk
**Calories, 1 crepe:** 75

*From Health Valley Foods.*

## Creamy Cranberry Sherbet

This super dessert looks like a little pink cloud dotted with bits of deep red.

| | | |
|---|---|---|
| 1 c. | water | 250 mL |
| 2 c. | cranberry juice cocktail | 500 mL |
| 1 c. | fresh cranberries, cleaned | 250 mL |
| 2 env. | unflavored gelatin | 2 env. |
| 1 c. | skim evaporated milk | 250 mL |
| 2 env. | aspartame sweetener | 2 env. |

Combine water, 1 c. (250 mL) of the cranberry juice cocktail, cranberries and gelatin in a small saucepan. Stir to mix slightly. Allow to rest for 5 minutes or until gelatin softens. Cook and stir over medium heat until cranberries have completely "popped." Remove from heat. Stir in remaining cranberry juice cocktail and evaporated milk. Add aspartame sweetener and stir thoroughly. Pour into metal tray, pan or bowl. Place in freezer until mixture forms crystals around the edge of the pan. Beat until creamy. Return to pan and freeze; stir occasionally.

**Yield:** 8 servings
**Exchange, 1 serving:** 1 fruit
**Calories, 1 serving:** 42

## Yogurt Tortoni

| | | |
|---|---|---|
| 2 8-oz. cartons | plain yogurt | 2 227-g cartons |
| 1 c. | applesauce | 250 mL |
| ½ t. | vanilla extract | 2 mL |
| ¾ c. | Kretschmer wheat germ | 190 mL |
| ⅓ c. | walnuts, finely chopped | 90 mL |
| 1 T. | honey | 15 mL |

Combine yogurt, applesauce and vanilla. Stir well to blend. Mix wheat germ, walnuts and honey together. Reserve ¼ c. (60 mL) wheat germ mixture for the topping. Add remaining wheat germ mixture to yogurt mixture. Blend well. Spoon into paper-lined muffin-pan cups. Top with reserved wheat germ mixture. Pat in lightly. Freeze for at least 2 hours or overnight. Let stand at room temperature for 15 to 20 minutes before serving.

**Yield:** 9 servings
**Exchange, 1 serving:** 1 bread, ⅕ fat
**Calories, 1 serving:** 84

*With the courtesy of Kretschmer Wheat Germ/International Multifoods.*

## Frosty Pineapple Dessert

| 20-oz. can | Featherweight water-pack | 600-g can |
| | pineapple chunks, drained | |
| 3½ c. | chopped ice | 875 mL |
| ½ t. | vanilla extract | 2 mL |
| dash | mint extract | dash |
| 6 | mint sprigs | 6 |

Combine all ingredients except the mint sprigs in a blender. Blend at high speed until finely crushed. Serve immediately in chilled dessert dishes with mint sprigs on top.

**Yield:** 6 servings
**Exchange, 1 serving:** 1 fruit
**Calories, 1 serving:** 50

*Based on a recipe from Featherweight Brand Foods.*

## Wheat Germ Single-Crust Pastry

| 1 c. | all-purpose flour | 25 mL |
| 2 T. | Kretschmer wheat germ | 30 mL |
| ½ t. | salt | 2 mL |
| 6 T. | vegetable shortening | 90 mL |
| 2–3 T. | cold water | 30–45 mL |

Combine flour, wheat germ and salt in bowl. Stir well to blend. Cut in shortening with pastry blender until mixture looks like coarse meal. Add water a little at a time, mixing lightly with fork. Shape dough into a firm ball. Refrigerate, it desired, for easier handling and to prevent shrinkage. Roll out into a 12-in. (30.5-cm) circle on a lightly floured cloth-covered board. Place loosely in 9-in. (23-cm) pie plate. Fold edge under. Press into upright rim. Flute as desired. Prick entire surface of pastry bottom and sides with fork before baking. Bake at 475 °F (250 °C) for 8 to 10 minutes until lightly browned. Cool on rack.

**Yield:** 9-in. (23-cm) piecrust or 8 servings
**Exchange, 1 serving:** 2 bread
**Calories, 1 serving:** 135

*With the courtesy of Kretschmer Wheat Germ/International Multifoods.*

## 100 Percent Whole Wheat Pastry

| 1 c. | whole wheat flour | 250 mL |
| ½ t. | salt | 2 mL |
| 6 T. | vegetable shortening | 90 mL |
| 2–3 T. | cold water | 30–40 mL |

Measure flour into a bowl and add salt. Stir to blend. Cut in half the shortening with a pastry blender until mixture looks like coarse meal, then the remaining shortening until particles are the size of small peas. Add water a little at a time, mixing lightly with a fork. Shape dough into a firm ball with hands. Flatten with your palm. Refrigerate, if desired, for easier handling and to prevent shrinkage. Roll out into a 12-in. (30.5-cm) circle on lightly floured cloth-covered board. Place loosely in 9-in. (23-cm) pie pan. Fold edge under. Press to make an upright rim. Flute edge, as desired. Prick entire surface of bottom and sides with a fork before baking pastry. Bake at 425 °F (220 °C) for 10 to 12 minutes. Cool on rack.

**Yield:** 9-in. (23-cm) piecrust or 8 servings
**Exchange, 1 serving:** 2 bread
**Calories, 1 serving:** 133

### Rye Pastry

| | | |
|---|---|---|
| 1¼ c. | *medium rye flour* | 310 mL |
| 1 t. | *granulated sugar replacement* | 5 mL |
| ½ t. | *baking powder* | 2 mL |
| ½ t. | *salt* | 2 mL |
| ⅓ c. | *vegetable shortening* | 90 mL |
| 3–4 T. | *cold water* | 45–60 mL |

Measure flour into a bowl and add the sugar, baking powder and salt. Stir well to blend. Cut in the shortening until mixture looks like coarse meal. Add water a little at a time, mixing lightly with fork. With your hands, shape dough into a firm ball. Roll into a 12-in. (30.5-cm) circle on lightly floured, cloth-covered board. Place loosely in a 9-in. (23-cm) pie pan. Fold edge under. Press to make an upright rim. Flute edge. Prick bottom and sides with a fork before baking pastry. Bake at 425 °F (220 °C) for 8 to 10 minutes. Cool on rack.

**Yield:** 9-in. (23-cm) piecrust or 8 servings
**Exchange, 1 serving:** 1 bread, 1½ fat
**Calories, 1 serving:** 132

### Lower-Calorie Pastry

| | | |
|---|---|---|
| ¾ c. | *zwieback crumbs* | 190 mL |
| 3 T. | *unsalted margarine, melted* | 45 mL |

Combine crumbs with margarine. Press into a 9-in. (23-cm) pie pan. Bake at 350 °F (175 °C) for 8 minutes. Cool thoroughly.

**Yield:** 8 servings
**Exchange, 1 serving:** 1 fat, ½ bread
**Calories, 1 serving:** 80

# Snacks

## Whole Wheat Pretzels

| | | |
|---|---|---|
| 1½ c. | all-purpose flour | 375 mL |
| 1 pkg. | active dry yeast | 1 pkg. |
| 3 T. | instant nonfat dry milk | 45 mL |
| 1 T. | granulated sugar replacement | 15 mL |
| 1½ t. | salt | 7 mL |
| 1 T. | margarine | 15 mL |
| 1 c. | hot tap water | 250 mL |
| 1½ c. | stone-ground whole wheat flour | 375 mL |
| 1 | egg white | 1 |
| 1 T. | water | 15 mL |
| | coarse salt | |

Measure 1 c. (250 mL) of the all-purpose flour in a large bowl. Add the undissolved yeast, dry milk, sugar and salt. Stir well to blend. Add margarine and hot water. Stir in the whole wheat flour. Gradually stir in remaining all-purpose flour to make a soft dough that leaves sides of the bowl. Add extra water, if needed. Turn out onto floured board. Knead 5 to 10 minutes or until dough is smooth and elastic. Cover and let rest 15 minutes on board.

Punch dough down. Roll into a 12-in. (30-cm) square. Cut into 24 strips. Roll each strip into a 14-in. (35-cm)-long rope. Shape into pretzels. Place on greased baking sheets. Let stand, uncovered, 2 minutes. Brush dough with egg white mixed with 1 T. (15 mL) water. Sprinkle with coarse salt. Bake at 350 °F (175 °C) for 18 to 20 minutes until lightly browned. Immediately remove from baking sheet. Serve warm.

**Yield:** 24 pretzels
**Exchange, 2 pretzels:** 1 bread
**Calories, 2 pretzels:** 80

## Spicy Walnuts

Although nuts are high in calories, sometimes a spicy or sweet nut makes a nice addition to a salad or vegetable, particularly to entice those who wouldn't otherwise eat fresh or cooked vegetables. You might try using some of these on a salad with just a sweetened cider vinegar dressing.

| | | |
|---|---|---|
| 2 c. | *walnuts, broken into pieces* | *500 mL* |
| ½ c. | *liquid sugar replacement* | *125 mL* |
| ¼ c. | *water* | *60 mL* |
| ½ t. | *orange rind, grated* | *2 mL* |
| ½ t. | *lemon rind, grated* | *2 mL* |
| ¼ t. | *ground cinnamon* | *1 mL* |
| ¼ t. | *ground ginger* | *1 mL* |
| *dash each* | *ground clove, nutmeg and allspice* | *dash each* |

Combine all ingredients in a saucepan. Cook and stir until liquid has evaporated. Spread nuts on a tabletop or baking sheet. Cool. Store in refrigerator or freezer.
**Yield:** 2 c. (500 mL)
**Exchange, 2 T. (30 mL):** 2 fat
**Calories, 2 T. (30 mL):** 92

## Salted Garbanzo Beans

A nice evening snack instead of popcorn.

| | | |
|---|---|---|
| 2 c. | *Jack Rabbit garbanzo beans (chick-peas)* | *500 mL* |
| 1 qt. | *water* | *1 L* |
| ¼ c. | *salt* | *60 mL* |
| | *shortening or oil for frying* | |

Combine water and salt in a saucepan. Cook and stir over medium heat until salt is completely dissolved. Add garbanzo beans. Simmer for 10 minutes. Remove pan from heat, cover and allow garbanzo beans to soak overnight. Drain and spread garbanzo beans out in a single layer to dry at room temperature; or pat dry with a towel. In a deep fryer, heat shortening or oil to 350 °F (175 °C). Fry a few at a time for 6 to 8 minutes. Drain on a paper towel
**Yield:** 3 c. (750 mL)
**Exchange, ¼ c. (60 mL):** 1 bread
**Calories, ¼ c. (60 mL):** 67

# Lazy-Day Pizza

**Crust**

| | | |
|---|---|---|
| 2 c. | graham flour | 500 mL |
| 1 pkg. | active dry yeast | 1 pkg. |
| ¾ t. | salt | 4 mL |
| 1 c. | hot tap water | 250 mL |
| 1 T. | vegetable oil | 15 mL |
| 1 T. | honey | 15 mL |

Measure flour into a large bowl. Add undissolved yeast and salt. Stir to blend. Add hot water, oil and honey. Stir vigorously until all ingredients are well mixed. Cover with plastic wrap and let rise for 10 minutes. Place dough on a greased pizza or other flat pan. Press dough to cover pan bottom and sides to form a rim. Reserve until ready to top with the sauce.

## PIZZA SAUCE

| | | |
|---|---|---|
| 15-oz. can | tomato sauce | 450-mL can |
| 1 t. | instant minced onion | 5 mL |
| ½ t. | oregano, crushed | 2 mL |
| ¼ t. | dried basil, crushed | 1 mL |
| ¼ t. | garlic powder | 1 mL |
| dash | pepper | dash |
| 1 lb. | lean ground beef, browned and drained | 500 g |
| 3-oz. can | mushroom pieces and stems | 90-g can |
| 8 oz. | mozzarella cheese, shredded | 240 g |
| ¼ c. | Parmesan cheese, grated | 60 mL |

Combine first 6 ingredients in a small bowl. Mix well. Spread sauce evenly on dough. Spoon beef on the sauce. Top with mushrooms and cheeses. Bake at 425 °F (220 °C) for 15 to 20 minutes until crust is golden brown and cheese melts.

**Yield:** 15 servings
**Exchange, 1 serving:** 1 bread, 1 high-fat meat
**Calories, 1 serving:** 172

## Stuffed Prunes

30 medium   dried prunes   30 medium
30 halves   English walnuts   30 halves

Wash prunes and soak overnight in water. Cook in the same water until prunes are semisoft but do not overcook. Drain thoroughly over a bowl. (You can refrigerate and use this liquid to sweeten other dishes; or chill and serve it as a beverage.) Remove stones from prunes. Place a half walnut in the cavity of each prune. Set on a rack and allow to dry slightly. Store in the refrigerator.

**Yield:** 30 snacks
**Exchange, 1 snack:** ½ fruit, ⅓ fat
**Calories, 1 snack:** 27

## Wheat Germ Granola

| | | |
|---|---|---|
| 3 c. | old-fashioned oatmeal | 750 mL |
| 1½ c. | wheat germ | 375 mL |
| ½ c. | almonds, chopped | 125 mL |
| ⅓ c. | sesame seeds | 90 mL |
| ¼ c. | vegetable oil | 60 mL |
| ⅓ c. | dietetic maple syrup | 90 mL |
| 1 c. | raisins | 250 mL |

Combine all ingredients except raisins, mixing well. Spread mixture evenly in a large shallow pan. Bake at 300 °F (150 °C) for 30 minutes, stirring every 10 minutes, until lightly toasted. Stir in the raisins. Cool completely. Store covered in a refrigerator.

**Yield:** 6½ cups (1625 mL)
**Exchange, ½ c. (125 mL):** 1 bread, 1 fruit, 1 fat
**Calories, ½ c. (125 mL):** 147

## Popcorn Variations

Popcorn is a very good fiber food. Here are a few variations you might like to try. I know each recipe makes a lot of popcorn, but popcorn freezes well after it is popped. All you have to do is store it in a freezer container.

| | | |
|---|---|---|
| 3.5-oz bag | *Pillsbury microwave frozen popcorn* | *99-g bag* |
| 2 T. | *any of the following seasonings or* | *30 mL* |
| | *a combination: taco seasoning mix,* | |
| | *creamy Italian salad dressing mix,* | |
| | *sweet-and-sour oriental seasoning mix,* | |
| | *nacho cheese sauce mix,* | |
| | *sloppy hot dog or hamburger* | |
| | *seasoning mix* | |

Pop the corn as directed on the package. Divide in half to make 4 c. (1 L) of popped corn in each half. Sprinkle 1 T. (15 mL) of your chosen seasoning mix over the popped corn you plan to serve. Shake or toss with a fork to completely coat. Reserve the remaining popped corn for future use.

**Yield:** 4 c. (1 L)
**Exchange, 1 c. (250 mL):** 1 bread
**Calories, 1 c. (250 mL):** 65

## Salted Pumpkin Seeds

I like to make these from the seeds of the Halloween pumpkin.

| | | |
|---|---|---|
| 2 c. | *water* | *500 mL* |
| ¼ c. | *salt* | *60 mL* |
| 2 c. | *pumpkin seeds* | *500mL* |

Combine water and salt in a saucepan. Cook and stir until salt dissolves; cool. Add pumpkin seeds and soak overnight. Drain thoroughly. Pat seeds dry with a paper towel. Place on a cookie sheet. Bake at 300 °F (150 °C) until seeds are dry, about 1 hour.

**Yield:** 2 c. (500 mL)
**Exchange, ¼ c. (60 mL):** 2 fat
**Calories, ¼ c. (60 mL):** 92

# ᴄAppendix

## Food Exchange Lists

If variety is the spice of life. Exchange Lists are just what you're looking for.

What do we mean by Exchange Lists? When we think of an "exchange" we automatically think of a "substitute" or a "trade." (I'll trade you an apple for an orange.) Basically, that's how it works, but the possibilities are endless.

Diets are sometimes stated in very dull, specific terms. For example:

| | |
|---|---|
| Orange juice | 1/2 cup |
| Oatmeal | 1/2 cup |
| Rye toast | 1 slice |
| Soft cooked egg | 1 |
| Butter | 1 teaspoon |
| Milk | 1/2 pint |

Exchange Lists take the dreariness out of diets. The Lists are groups of measured foods of the same value that can be substituted in Meal Plans. Foods have been divided into six groups, or Exchanges. For example, vegetables are listed in one group and fats are listed in another group. Foods in any *one group* can be substituted or exchanged with other foods in the *same group*.

Within each group an Exchange is approximately equal in calories and in the amount of carbohydrate, protein and fat. In addition, each Exchange contains similar minerals and vitamins.

The number of calories in any food expresses the energy value of the food. As an adult you may need fewer calories to maintain normal weight. Many people as they reach their 30's and 40's become physically less active but do not change their eating habits. They store their excess calories as fat. The result: the famous "middle age spread." Your diet counselor will know how many calories you require each day to maintain good health.

Fats, carbohydrates and proteins are the three major energy sources in foods. The most common carbohydrates are sugars and starches. Proteins yield energy and contain nitrogen, which is essential for life. Fats provide energy and are the most concentrated source of calories. Alcohol also contributes calories.

Minerals and vitamins are substances present in food in small amounts and perform essential functions in the body. The foods of each Exchange make a specific nutritional contribution. No one Exchange group can supply all the nutrients needed for a well-balanced diet. It takes all six of them working together as a team to supply your nutritional needs for good health.

The exchange lists are based on material in *Exchange Lists for Meal Planning* prepared by Committees of the American Diabetes Association, Inc., and the American Dietetic Association in cooperation with the National Institute of Arthritis, Metabolism and Digestive Diseases and the National Heart and Lung Institute, National Institutes of Health, Public Health Service, U.S. Department of Health, Education and Welfare.

# LIST 1 — Milk Exchanges (Includes **Non-Fat** Low-Fat and Whole Milk)

One Exchange of Milk contains 12 grams of carbohydrate, 8 grams of protein, a trace of fat and 80 calories.

Milk is a basic food for your Meal Plan for very good reasons. Milk is the leading source of calcium. It is a good source of phosphorus, protein, some of the B-complex vitamins, including folacin and vitamin $B_{12}$, and vitamins A and D. Magnesium is also found in milk.

Since it is a basic ingredient in many recipes you will not find it difficult to include milk in your Meal Plan. Milk can be used not only to drink but can be added to cereal, coffee, tea and other foods.

This List shows the kinds and amounts of milk or milk products to use for one Milk Exchange. Those which appear in **bold type** are **non-fat**. Low-Fat and Whole Milk contain saturated fat.

### Non-Fat Fortified Milk

| | |
|---|---|
| **Skim or non-fat milk** | 1 cup |
| **Powdered (non-fat dry, before adding liquid)** | 1/3 cup |
| **Canned, evaporated – skim milk** | 1/2 cup |
| **Buttermilk made from skim milk** | 1 cup |
| **Yogurt made from skim milk (plain, unflavored)** | 1 cup |

### Low-Fat Fortified Milk

| | |
|---|---|
| 1% fat fortified milk (omit 1/2 Fat Exchange) | 1 cup |
| 2% fat fortified milk (omit 1 Fat Exchange) | 1 cup |
| Yogurt made from 2% fortified milk (plain, unflavored) (omit 1 Fat Exchange) | 1 cup |

### Whole Milk (Omit 2 Fat Exchanges)

| | |
|---|---|
| Whole milk | 1 cup |
| Canned, evaporated whole milk | 1/2 cup |
| Buttermilk made from whole milk | 1 cup |
| Yogurt made from whole milk (plain, unflavored) | 1 cup |

# LIST 2 — Vegetable Exchanges

One Exchange of Vegetables contains about 5 grams of carbohydrate, 2 grams of protein and 25 calories.

The generous use of many vegetables, served either alone or in other foods such as casseroles, soups or salads, contributes to sound health and vitality.

Dark green and deep yellow vegetables are among the leading sources of vitamin A. Many of the vegetables in this group are notable sources of vitamin C — asparagus, broccoli, brussels sprouts, cabbage, cauliflower, collards, kale, dandelion, mustard and turnip greens, spinach, rutabagas, to tomatoes and turnips. A number, including broccoli, brussels sprouts, beet greens, chard and tomato juice, are particularly good sources of potassium. High folacin values are found in asparagus, beets, broccoli, brussels sprouts, cauliflower, collards, kale and lettuce. Moderate amounts of vitamin $B_6$ are supplied by broccoli, brussels sprouts, cauliflower, collards, spinach, sauerkraut and tomatoes and tomato juice. Fiber is present in all vegetables.

Whether you serve them cooked or raw, wash all vegetables even though they look clean. If fat is added in the preparation, omit the equivalent number of Fat Exchanges. The average amount of fat contained in a Vegetable Exchange that is cooked with fat meat or other fats is one Fat Exchange.

This List shows the kinds of **vegetables** to use for one Vegetable Exchange. One Exchange is ½ cup.

| | |
|---|---|
| **Asparagus** | **Greens:** |
| **Bean Sprouts** | **Mustard** |
| **Beets** | **Spinach** |
| **Broccoli** | **Turnip** |
| **Brussels Sprouts** | **Mushrooms** |
| **Cabbage** | **Okra** |
| **Carrots** | **Onions** |
| **Cauliflower** | **Rhubarb** |
| **Celery** | **Rutabaga** |
| **Eggplant** | **Sauerkraut** |
| **Green Pepper** | **String Beans, green or yellow** |
| **Greens:** | **Summer Squash** |
| **Beet** | **Tomatoes** |
| **Chards** | **Tomato Juice** |
| **Collards** | **Turnips** |
| **Dandelion** | **Vegetable Juice Cocktail** |
| **Kale** | **Zucchini** |

The following **raw vegetables** may be used as desired:

| | |
|---|---|
| **Chicory** | **Lettuce** |
| **Chinese Cabbage** | **Parsley** |
| **Cucumbers** | **Pickles, Dill** |
| **Endive** | **Radishes** |
| **Escarole** | **Watercress** |

**Starchy Vegetables** are found in the Bread Exchange List.

**LIST** 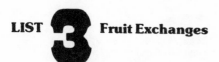 **Fruit Exchanges**

One Exchange of Fruit contains 10 grams of carbohydrate and 40 calories.

Everyone likes to buy fresh fruits when they are in the height of their season. But you can also buy fresh fruits and can or freeze them for off-season use. For variety serve fruit as a salad or in combination with other foods for dessert.

Fruits are valuable for vitamins, minerals and fiber. Vitamin C is abundant in citrus fruits and fruit juices and is found in raspberries, strawberries, mangoes, cantaloupes, honeydews and papayas. The better sources of vitamin A among these fruits include fresh or dried apricots, mangoes, cantaloupes, nectarines, yellow peaches and persimmons. Oranges, orange juice and cantaloupe provide more folacin than most of the other fruits in this listing. Many fruits are a valuable source of potassium, especially apricots, bananas, several of the berries, grapefruit, grapefruit juice, mangoes, cantaloupes, honeydews, nectarines, oranges, orange juice and peaches.

Fruit may be used fresh, dried, canned or frozen, cooked or raw, as long as no sugar is added.

This List shows the kinds and amounts of **fruits** to use for one Fruit Exchange.

| | | | |
|---|---|---|---|
| **Apple** | 1 small | **Apricots, fresh** | 2 medium |
| **Apple Juice** | 1/3 cup | **Apricots, dried** | 4 halves |
| **Applesauce (unsweetened)** | 1/2 cup | **Banana** | 1/2 small |

| Berries | | Honeydew | 1/8 medium |
|---|---|---|---|
| **Blackberries** | 1/2 cup | **Watermelon** | 1 cup |
| **Blueberries** | 1/2 cup | **Nectarine** | 1 small |
| **Raspberries** | 1/2 cup | **Orange** | 1 small |
| **Strawberries** | 3/4 cup | **Orange Juice** | 1/2 cup |
| Cherries | 10 large | **Papaya** | 3/4 cup |
| Cider | 1/3 cup | **Peach** | 1 medium |
| Dates | 2 | **Pear** | 1 small |
| Figs, fresh | 1 | **Persimmon, native** | 1 medium |
| Figs, dried | 1 | **Pineapple** | 1/2 cup |
| Grapefruit | 1/2 | **Pineapple Juice** | 1/3 cup |
| Grapefruit Juice | 1/2 cup | **Plums** | 2 medium |
| Grapes | 12 | **Prunes** | 2 medium |
| Grape Juice | 1/4 cup | **Prune Juice** | 1/4 cup |
| Mango | 1/2 small | **Raisins** | 2 tablespoons |
| Melon | | **Tangerine** | 1 medium |
| Cantaloupe | 1/4 small | | |

**Cranberries** may be used as desired if no sugar is added.

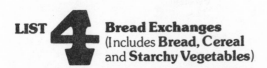

**LIST 4** **Bread Exchanges**
(Includes **Bread, Cereal** and **Starchy Vegetables**)

One Exchange of Bread contains 15 grams of carbohydrate, 2 grams of protein and 70 calories.

In this List, whole-grain and enriched breads and cereals, germ and bran products and dried beans and peas are good sources of iron and among the better sources of thiamin. The whole-grain, bran and germ products have more fiber than products made from refined flours. Dried beans and peas are also good sources of fiber. Wheat germ, bran, dried beans, potatoes, lima beans, parsnips, pumpkin and winter squash are particularly good sources of potassium. The better sources of folacin in this listing include whole-wheat bread, wheat germ, dried beans, corn, lima beans, parsnips, green peas, pumpkin and sweet potato.

Starchy vegetables are included in this List, because they contain the same amount of carbohydrate and protein as one slice of bread.

This List shows the kinds and amounts of **Breads, Cereals, Starchy Vegetables** and Prepared Foods to use for one Bread Exchange. Those which appear in **bold type** are **low-fat.**

**Bread**

| | | | |
|---|---|---|---|
| **White (including French and Italian)** | 1 slice | **Puffed Cereal (unfrosted)** | 1 cup |
| | | **Cereal (cooked)** | 1/2 cup |
| | | **Grits (cooked)** | 1/2 cup |
| **Whole Wheat** | 1 slice | **Rice or Barley (cooked)** | 1/2 cup |
| **Rye or Pumpernickel** | 1 slice | **Pasta (cooked),** | 1/2 cup |
| **Raisin** | 1 slice | **Spaghetti, Noodles,** | |
| **Bagel, small** | 1/2 | **Macaroni** | |
| **English Muffin, small** | 1/2 | **Popcorn (popped, no fat** | 3 cups |
| **Plain Roll, bread** | 1 | **added, large kernel)** | |
| **Frankfurter Roll** | 1/2 | **Cornmeal (dry)** | 2 Tbs. |
| **Hamburger Bun** | 1/2 | **Flour** | 2-1/2 Tbs. |
| **Dried Bread Crumbs** | 3 Tbs. | **Wheat Germ** | 1/4 cup |
| **Tortilla, 6"** | 1 | **Crackers** | |

**Cereal**

| | | | |
|---|---|---|---|
| **Bran Flakes** | 1/2 cup | **Arrowroot** | 3 |
| **Other ready-to-eat** | | **Graham, 2-1/2" sq.** | 2 |
| **unsweetened Cereal** | 3/4 cup | **Matzoth, 4" x 6"** | 1/2 |
| | | **Oyster** | 20 |

| | | |
|---|---|---|
| **Pretzels, 3-1/8" long x 1/8" dia.** | 25 | |
| **Rye Wafers, 2" x 3-1/2"** | 3 | |
| **Saltines** | 6 | |
| **Soda, 2-1/2" sq.** | 4 | |

**Dried Beans, Peas and Lentils**

| | |
|---|---|
| **Beans, Peas, Lentils (dried and cooked)** | 1/2 cup |
| **Baked Beans, no pork (canned)** | 1/4 cup |

**Starchy Vegetables**

| | |
|---|---|
| **Corn** | 1/3 cup |
| **Corn on Cob** | 1 small |
| **Lima Beans** | 1/2 cup |
| **Parsnips** | 2/3 cup |
| **Peas, Green (canned or frozen)** | 1/2 cup |
| **Potato, White** | 1 small |
| **Potato (mashed)** | 1/2 cup |
| **Pumpkin** | 3/4 cup |
| **Winter Squash, Acorn or Butternut** | 1/2 cup |
| **Yam or Sweet Potato** | 1/4 cup |

Prepared Foods

| | |
|---|---|
| Biscuit 2" dia. (omit 1 Fat Exchange) | 1 |
| Corn Bread, 2" x 2" x 1" (omit 1 Fat Exchange) | 1 |
| Corn Muffin, 2" dia. (omit 1 Fat Exchange) | 1 |
| Crackers, round butter type (omit 1 Fat Exchange) | 5 |
| Muffin, plain small (omit 1 Fat Exchange) | 1 |
| Potatoes, French Fried, length 2" to 3-1/2" (omit 1 Fat Exchange) | 8 |
| Potato or Corn Chips (omit 2 Fat Exchanges) | 15 |
| Pancake, 5" x 1/2" (omit 1 Fat Exchange) | 1 |
| Waffle, 5" x 1/2" (omit 1 Fat Exchange) | 1 |

## LIST 5   Meat Exchanges    Lean Meat

One Exchange of Lean Meat (1 oz.) contains 7 grams of protein, 3 grams of fat and 55 calories.

---

All of the foods in the Meat Exchange Lists are good sources of protein and many are also good sources of iron, zinc, vitamin $B_{12}$ (present only in foods of animal origin) and other vitamins of the vitamin B-complex.

Cholesterol is of animal origin. Foods of plant origin have no cholesterol.

Oysters are outstanding for their high content of zinc. Crab, liver, trimmed lean meats, the dark muscle meat of turkey, dried beans and peas and peanut butter all have much less zinc than oysters but are still good sources.

Dried beans, peas and peanut butter are particularly good sources of magnesium; also potassium.

Your choice of meat groups through the week will depend on your blood lipid values. Consult with your diet counselor and your physician regarding your selection.

You may use the meat, fish or other Meat Exchanges that are prepared for the family when no fat or flour has been added. If meat is fried, use the fat included in the Meal Plan. Meat juices with the fat removed may be used with your meat or vegetables for added flavor. **Be certain to trim off all visible fat** and measure after it has been cooked. A three-ounce serving of cooked meat is about equal to four ounces of raw meat.

To plan a diet low in saturated fat and cholesterol, choose only those Exchanges in **bold type**.

This List shows the kinds and amounts of **Lean Meat** and other Protein-Rich Foods to use for one Low-Fat Meat Exchange. **Trim off all visible fat.**

| | | |
|---|---|---|
| **Beef:** | **Baby Beef (very lean), Chipped Beef, Chuck, Flank Steak, Tenderloin, Plate Ribs, Plate Skirt Steak, Round (bottom, top), All cuts Rump, Spare Ribs, Tripe** | 1 oz. |
| **Lamb:** | **Leg, Rib, Sirloin, Loin (roast and chops), Shank, Shoulder** | 1 oz. |
| **Pork:** | **Leg (Whole Rump, Center Shank), Ham, Smoked (center slices)** | 1 oz. |
| **Veal:** | **Leg, Loin, Rib, Shank, Shoulder, Cutlets** | 1 oz. |

**Poultry: Meat** <u>without skin</u> **of Chicken, Turkey, Cornish Hen,**   1 oz.
   **Guinea Hen, Pheasant**
**Fish:**  **Any fresh or frozen**                                         1 oz.
      **Canned Salmon, Tuna, Mackerel, Crab and Lobster,**               1/4 cup
      **Clams, Oysters, Scallops, Shrimp,**                              5 or 1 oz.
      **Sardines, drained**                                              3
**Cheeses containing less than 5% butterfat**                            1 oz.
**Cottage Cheese, Dry and 2% butterfat**                                 1/4 cup
**Dried Beans and Peas (omit 1 Bread Exchange)**                         1/2 cup

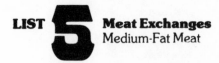

**LIST**  **Meat Exchanges**
Medium-Fat Meat

One Exhange of Medium-Fat Meat (1 oz.) contains 7 grams of protein, 5 grams of fat and 75 calories.

This List shows the kinds and amounts of Medium-Fat Meat and other Protein-Rich Foods to use for one Medium-Fat Meat Exchange. **Trim off all visible fat.**

Beef:   Ground (15% fat), Corned Beef (canned), Rib Eye, Round   1 oz.
      (ground commercial)
Pork:   Loin (all cuts Tenderloin), Shoulder Arm (picnic), Shoulder Blade,   1 oz.
      Boston Butt, Canadian Bacon, Boiled Ham
Liver, Heart, Kidney and Sweetbreads (these are high in cholesterol)   1 oz.
Cottage Cheese, creamed                                                 1/4 cup
Cheese: Mozzarella, Ricotta, Farmer's cheese, Neufchatel,               1 oz.
      Parmesan                                                          3 tbs.
Egg (high in cholesterol)                                               1
**Peanut Butter** (omit 2 additional Fat Exchanges)                     2 tbs.

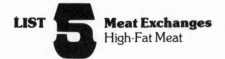

**LIST**  **Meat Exchanges**
High-Fat Meat

One Exchange of High-Fat Meat (1 oz.) contains 7 grams of protein, 8 grams of fat and 100 calories.

This List shows the kinds and amounts of High-Fat Meat and other Protein-Rich Foods to use for one High-Fat Meat Exchange. **Trim off all visible fat.**

Beef:   Brisket, Corned Beef (Brisket), Ground Beef (more than   1 oz.
      20% fat), Hamburger (commercial), Chuck (ground
      commercial), Roasts (Rib), Steaks (Club and Rib)
Lamb:   Breast                                                          1 oz.
Pork:   Spare Ribs, Loin (Back Ribs), Pork (ground), Country style   1 oz.
      Ham, Deviled Ham
Veal:   Breast                                                          1 oz.
Poultry: Capon, Duck (domestic), Goose                                  1 oz.
Cheese: Cheddar Types                                                   1 oz.
Cold Cuts                                                               4-1/2"x 1/8" slice
Frankfurter                                                             1 small

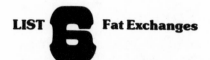

**LIST 6**   **Fat Exchanges**

One Exchange of Fat contains
5 grams of fat and 45 calories.

Fats are of both animal and vegetable origin and range from liquid oils to hard fats.

Oils are fats that remain liquid at room temperature and are usually of vegetable origin. Common fats obtained from vegetables are corn oil, olive oil and peanut oil. Some of the common animal fats are butter and bacon fat.

Since all fats are concentrated sources of calories, foods on this List should be measured carefully to control weight. Margarine, butter, cream and cream cheese contain vitamin A. Use the fats on this List in the amounts on the Meal Plan.

This List shows the kinds and amounts of Fat-Containing Foods to use for one Fat Exchange. To plan a diet low in Saturated Fat select only those Exchanges which appear in **bold type**. They are **Polyunsaturated.**

| | |
|---|---|
| **Margarine, soft, tub or stick***  | 1 teaspoon |
| **Avocado (4" in diameter)****  | 1/8 |
| **Oil, Corn, Cottonseed, Safflower,** | |
| **Soy, Sunflower** | 1 teaspoon |
| **Oil, Olive**** | 1 teaspoon |
| **Oil, Peanut**** | 1 teaspoon |
| **Olives**** | 5 small |
| **Almonds**** | 10 whole |
| **Pecans**** | 2 large whole |
| **Peanuts**** | |
| **Spanish** | 20 whole |
| **Virginia** | 10 whole |
| **Walnuts** | 6 small |
| **Nuts, other**** | 6 small |
| | |
| Margarine, regular stick | 1 teaspoon |
| Butter | 1 teaspoon |
| Bacon fat | 1 teaspoon |
| Bacon, crisp | 1 strip |
| Cream, light | 2 tablespoons |
| Cream, sour | 2 tablespoons |
| Cream, heavy | 1 tablespoon |
| Cream Cheese | 1 tablespoon |
| French dressing*** | 1 tablespoon |
| Italian dressing*** | 1 tablespoon |
| Lard | 1 teaspoon |
| Mayonnaise*** | 1 teaspoon |
| Salad dressing, mayonnaise type*** | 2 teaspoons |
| Salt pork | 3/4 inch cube |

*Made with corn, cottonseed, safflower, soy or sunflower oil only
**Fat content is primarily monounsaturated
***If made with corn, cottonseed, safflower, soy or sunflower oil can be used on fat modified diet

# A Note on Products

Manufacturers contributing recipes to this book include the following information for your convenience. These companies developed the recipes for a general audience interested in high-fiber diet and I calculated the recipes for diabetics.

## ARNOLD FOODS COMPANY, INC.

1. Stone-Buhr® is a registered trademark of Arnold Foods Company, Inc.
2. Oroweat® and Northridge® are registered trademarks of Oroweat Foods Company.

> Arnold Foods Company, Inc.
> Suite 122
> 2001 Killebrew Drive
> Bloomington, MN 55420-1673

## THE ESTEE CORPORATION

Estee Corporation manufactures a wide variety of products made without ordinary table sugar and salt; many are low- or reduced-calorie products. These products are available nationally in the diet department of supermarket chains and independent stores and by mail order.

Consumers can send for nutrition and diabetic exchange information, recipes and label reading guide by writing to

> The Estee Corporation
> Consumer Relations
> 169 Lackawanna Avenue
> Parsippany, NJ 07054

## FEATHERWEIGHT

Featherweight® offers over 150 products specially designed to meet the requirements of consumers on medically-directed diets. For coupons and additional information write to

> Featherweight®
> Sandoz Nutrition Corporation
> P.O. Box 370
> Minneapolis, MN 55440

## INTERNATIONAL MULTIFOODS

For additional product or recipe information for Kretschmer Wheat Germ or Robin Hood Flour, write to

> Consumer Communications
> International Multifoods
> Multifoods Tower, Box 2942
> Minneapolis, MN 55402

## KELLOGG COMPANY

Kellogg's All-Bran® and Bran Buds® are registered trademarks belonging to the Kellogg Company.

> Kellogg Company
> Battle Creek, MI 49016

## THE PILLSBURY COMPANY

"Nutrition information for Pillsbury products is current as of 1984. Because it can vary from time to time, please consult the product's label before purchase."

> The Pillsbury Company
> MS 3726
> Minneapolis MN 55402

# Index